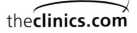
the**clinics**.com

VETERINARY CLINICS
OF NORTH AMERICA

Small Animal Practice

General Orthopedics

GUEST EDITOR
Walter C. Renberg, DVM, MS

September 2005 • Volume 35 • Number 5

SAUNDERS

An Imprint of Elsevier, Inc.
PHILADELPHIA   LONDON   TORONTO   MONTREAL   SYDNEY   TOKYO

W.B. SAUNDERS COMPANY
A Division of Elsevier Inc.

Elsevier, Inc., 1600 John F. Kennedy Blvd., Suite 1800, Philadelphia, PA 19103-2899

http://www.vetsmall.theclinics.com

VETERINARY CLINICS OF NORTH AMERICA:
SMALL ANIMAL PRACTICE
September 2005
Editor: John Vassallo

Volume 35, Number 5
ISSN 0195-5616
ISBN 1-4160-2847-1

The ideas and opinions expressed in *Veterinary Clinics of North America: Small Animal Practice* do not necessarily reflect those of the Publisher. The Publisher does not assume any responsibility for any injury and/or damage to persons or property arising out of or related to any use of the material contained in this periodical. The reader is advised to check the appropriate medical literature and the product information currently provided by the manufacturer of each drug to be administered to verify the dosage, the method and duration of administration, or contraindications. It is the responsibility of the treating physician or other health care professional, relying on independent experience and knowledge of the patient, to determine drug dosages and the best treatment for the patient. Mention of any product in this issue should not be construed as endorsement by the contributors, editors, or the Publisher of the product or manufacturers' claims.

Veterinary Clinics of North America: Small Animal Practice (ISSN 0195-5616) is published bimonthly (For Post Office use only: volume 35 issue 5 of 6) by Elsevier, Inc. Corporate and editorial offices: Elsevier, Inc., 1600 John F. Kennedy Blvd., Suite 1800, Philadelphia, PA 19103-2899. Accounting and circulation offices: 6277 Sea Harbor Drive, Orlando, FL 32887-4800. Periodicals postage paid at Orlando, FL 32862, and additional mailing offices. Subscription prices are $170.00 per year for US individuals, $260.00 per year for US institutions, $85.00 per year for US students and residents, $215.00 per year for Canadian individuals, $325.00 per year for Canadian institutions, $225.00 per year for international individuals, $325.00 per year for international institutions and $113.00 per year for Canadian and foreign students/residents. To receive student/resident rate, orders must be accompanied by name of affiliated institution, date of term, and the *signature* of program/residency coordinator on institution letterhead. Orders will be billed at individual rate until proof of status is received. Foreign air speed delivery is included in all *Clinics* subscription prices. All prices are subject to change without notice. POSTMASTER: Send address changes to *Veterinary Clinics of North America: Small Animal Practice*, Elsevier, Customer Service Department, 6277 Sea Harbor Drive, Orlando, FL 32887-4800, USA; phone: (+1)(877) 839-7126 [toll free number for US customers], or (+1)(407) 345-4020 [customers outside US]; fax: (+1)(407) 363-1354; email: usjcs@elsevier.com

Veterinary Clinics of North America: Small Animal Practice is also published in Japanese by Gakusosha Company Ltd., 2-16-28 Nishikata, Bunkyo-ku, Tokyo 113, Japan.

Reprints: For copies of 100 or more, of articles in this publication, please contact the Commercial Reprints Department, Elsevier Inc., 360 Park Avenue South, New York, New York 10010-1710. Tel. (212) 633-3813 Fax: (212) 462-1935, email: reprints@elsevier.com

Veterinary Clinics of North America: Small Animal Practice is covered in *Current Contents/Agriculture, Biology and Environmental Sciences, Science Citation Index, ASCA, Index Medicus, Excerpta Medica, and BIOSIS*.

Printed in the United States of America.

VETERINARY CLINICS
SMALL ANIMAL PRACTICE

General Orthopedics

GUEST EDITOR

WALTER C. RENBERG, DVM, MS, Diplomate, American College of Veterinary Surgeons; Associate Professor, Small Animal Surgery, Department of Clinical Sciences, College of Veterinary Medicine, Kansas State University, Manhattan, Kansas

CONTRIBUTORS

JUDE T. BORDELON, DVM, Resident, Small Animal Surgery, Department of Veterinary Clinical Sciences, College of Veterinary Medicine, Oklahoma State University, Stillwater, Oklahoma

LORETTA J. BUBENIK, DVM, MS, Diplomate, American College of Veterinary Surgeons; Assistant Professor, Companion Animal Surgery, Veterinary Clinical Sciences, Louisiana State University School of Veterinary Medicine, Baton Rouge, Louisiana

RUTHANNE CHUN, DVM, Diplomate, American College of Veterinary Internal Medicine (Oncology); Clinical Associate Professor, University of Wisconsin-Madison, Madison, Wisconsin

MICHAEL G. CONZEMIUS, DVM, PhD, Diplomate, American College of Veterinary Surgeons; Associate Professor of Small Animal Surgery, College of Veterinary Medicine, Iowa State University, Ames, Iowa

JENNIFER DEMKO, DVM, Small Animal Intern, Department of Clinical Sciences, College of Veterinary Medicine, Mississippi State University, Mississippi State, Mississippi

MARIA A. FAHIE, DVM, MS, Diplomate, American College of Veterinary Surgeons; Associate Professor, Small Animal Surgery, College of Veterinary Medicine, Western University of Health Sciences, Pomona, California

RON McLAUGHLIN, DVM, DVSc, Diplomate, American College of Veterinary Surgeons; Associate Professor and Chief, Small Animal Surgery, Department of Clinical Sciences, College of Veterinary Medicine, Mississippi State University, Mississippi State, Mississippi

H. FULTON REAUGH, DVM, Resident, Small Animal Surgery, Department of Veterinary Clinical Sciences, College of Veterinary Medicine, Oklahoma State University, Stillwater, Oklahoma

WALTER C. RENBERG, DVM, MS, Diplomate, American College of Veterinary Surgeons; Associate Professor, Small Animal Surgery, Department of Clinical Sciences, College of Veterinary Medicine, Kansas State University, Manhattan, Kansas

MARK C. ROCHAT, DVM, MS, Diplomate, American College of Veterinary Surgeons; Professor and Chief, Small Animal Surgery, Department of Veterinary Clinical Sciences, Center for Veterinary Health Sciences, Oklahoma State University, Stillwater, Oklahoma

JAMES K. ROUSH, DVM, MS, Diplomate, American College of Veterinary Surgeons; Professor and Section Head, Small Animal Surgery, Department of Clinical Sciences, College of Veterinary Medicine, Kansas State University, Manhattan, Kansas

JENNIFER VANDERVOORT, DVM, Resident in Small Animal Surgery, College of Veterinary Medicine, Iowa State University, Ames, Iowa

VETERINARY CLINICS
SMALL ANIMAL PRACTICE

General Orthopedics

CONTENTS

VOLUME 35 • NUMBER 5 • SEPTEMBER 2005

Fracture repair in small animals has arrived at a crossroads because of advances in fracture repair and client demands. Research into bone healing and repair techniques, collective professional experience, economics, and client demands are obligating veterinarians to greater expertise in the actual act of repairing fractures. The influx of surgery specialists into burgeoning private practices has improved access to specialty service beyond what the limited number of academic practices could previously provide and has raised the local standard of practice for orthopedic surgery at the same time. The necessity to deal with the preoperative and postoperative management of traumatized small animals by the general practitioner has not changed, however. Treatment of the small animal patient with a fractured bone does involve accurate definition of the fracture, selection of an appropriate method of fracture fixation from the variety of devices available, and correct application of the fixation. Far more than these, however, it involves assessment and treatment of the traumatized patient as a whole, including preanesthetic evaluation of critical body systems, preoperative preparation of the patient and client, and postoperative management of the repaired fracture and patient.

Malignancies of the musculoskeletal system in dogs and cats can be categorized as either primary or metastatic within the bony or soft structures that comprise the musculoskeletal system. By far, the most common tumor that affects the musculoskeletal system in dogs is osteosarcoma. The most common tumors that affect the musculoskeletal system in cats are injection site sarcomas. These tumors are locally infiltrative; whereas up to 25% metastasize, most animals die from our inability to control local disease. The aim of this article is to provide a brief review of the biologic behavior of and treatment recommendations for common tumors of the musculoskeletal system, excluding the oral and nasal cavities.

Traumatic luxation of joints of the appendicular skeleton is common. Timely and accurate identification of the luxation is essential to restoring normal function. Physical examination and radiographic assessment are commonly utilized for accurate identification and categorization. Conservative and surgical techniques are employed for treatment of luxations solely and in combination. Selection of appropriate reparative techniques is dependent on the joint injured as well as on other joint- and injury-specific factors.

Management of tendon conditions can be frustrating due to difficulty with diagnosis, choice of treatment or repair technique, prolonged tissue healing, and potential for permanent compromise of limb function after surgery. This article reviews tendon healing and reported tendon conditions, focusing on bicipital tenosynovitis and common calcaneal tendon injuries. Surgical management options, research in enhancement of tendon healing, and postoperative rehabilitation are also reviewed.

Total joint replacement has evolved over the past 50 years from a concept that was first attempted in people suffering from osteoarthritis to a commonly applied practice in veterinary medicine. Although many questions have been answered, several controversies still exist, with many implant and technical options being explored. Currently, total hip and elbow replacement are commercially available options viable for use in dogs. These options are detailed in this article. Joint replacement for other canine joints (ie, knee, hock, shoulder) that develop osteoarthritis likely will be developed in the near future.

Most orthopedic conditions that affect dogs are well described established conditions. Often, the current literature is focused on refinements in diagnosis, treatment, and management of these conditions. Improvement in worldwide reporting of emerging conditions offers veterinarians a greater awareness of new conditions as they occur. This article compiles into a single source what has been reported for five newly described disorders.

GOAL STATEMENT

The goal of the *Veterinary Clinics of North America: Small Animal Practice* is to keep practicing veterinarians up to date with current clinical practice in small animal medicine by providing timely articles reviewing the state of the art in small animal care.

ACCREDITATION

The *Veterinary Clinics of North America: Small Animal Practice* offers continuing education credits, awarded by Cummings School of Veterinary Medicine at Tufts University, Office of Continuing Education.

Cummings School of Veterinary Medicine at Tufts University is a designated provider of continuing veterinary medical education. Veterinarians participating in this learning activity may earn up to 6 credits per issue up to a maximum of 36 credits per year. Credits awarded may not apply toward license renewal in all states. It is the responsibility of each participant to verify the requirements of their state licensing board.

Credit can be earned by reading the text material, taking the examination online at *http://www.theclinics.com/home/cme*, and completing the program evaluation. Following your completion of the test and program evaluation, and review of any and all incorrect answers, you may print your certificate.

TO ENROLL

To enroll in the *Veterinary Clinics of North America: Small Animal Practice* Continuing Veterinary Medical Education Program, call customer service at 1-800-654-2452 or sign up online at *http://www.theclinics.com/home/cme*. The CVME program is now available at a special introductory rate of $99.95 for a year's subscription.

VETERINARY CLINICS
SMALL ANIMAL PRACTICE

ELSEVIER
SAUNDERS

Vet Clin Small Anim 35 (2005) xi–xii

VETERINARY CLINICS
SMALL ANIMAL PRACTICE

PREFACE

General Orthopedics

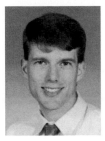

Walter C. Renberg, DVM, MS

Guest Editor

This issue of the *Veterinary Clinics of North America: Small Animal Practice* reviews the basic topic of small animal orthopedics. Orthopedic disease is an immense topic, and the discussion can be very complex. Subsequently, the concepts are difficult to cover adequately in a given forum and can be frustrating for the practitioner to review efficiently. Our hope is to partially fill the gap between large textbooks and journal articles. The former are capable of covering a wide variety of topics, but may become dated and suffer from having to balance detail on a given concept with the length of each section. The latter are generally current and detailed, but are specific enough to not be an efficient review source for many veterinarians. Our hope is that this issue falls somewhere in the middle–providing sufficiently detailed information on a good number of topics. We hope that we can provide an update and a review for the practitioner who has a genuine interest in staying current with orthopedic disease management.

The articles in this issue have been selected to cover the most commonly encountered orthopedic diseases as well as to touch upon new or often-confusing topics. We begin with a review of bone healing, arthritis, and bone infections, then discuss developmental diseases and fracture management. These are broad categories that most readers are familiar with in some ways. The articles discuss newer findings and highlight points that readers will find helpful as they review. The articles that follow–neoplasia, luxations, and tendon disease–are discussions of specific orthopedic ailments commonly encountered by the small animal practitioner. Finally, articles on joint

0195-5616/05/$ – see front matter
doi:10.1016/j.cvsm.2005.07.001

replacement and new diseases are designed to bring readers up-to-date with the latest developments in the field.

The authors hope that the readers will find this issue to be a useful tool in learning about orthopedic topics they have not pursued and to inspire them to review developments in areas in which they may feel a little rusty. The references point readers to more detailed coverage.

As Guest Editor, I sincerely appreciate the efforts of the authors who have contributed to this issue. Their shared experience and knowledge is an invaluable resource. I also express my thanks to Elsevier for allowing me this opportunity to share information with my colleagues in the veterinary profession.

Walter C. Renberg, DVM, MS
Department of Clinical Sciences
College of Veterinary Medicine
Kansas State University
1800 Denison Road
Manhattan, KS 66506, USA

E-mail address: renberg@vet.k-state.edu

Vet Clin Small Anim 35 (2005) 1073–1091

VETERINARY CLINICS
SMALL ANIMAL PRACTICE

Pathophysiology and Management of Arthritis

Walter C. Renberg, DVM, MS

Department of Clinical Sciences, College of Veterinary Medicine, Kansas State University, 1800 Denison Avenue, Manhattan, KS 66506, USA

U nderstanding and managing arthritis in veterinary patients are of great importance. Arthritis occupies a significant place in the public's mind and a larger place in the veterinarian's professional experiences. Aside from long bone fractures, most of the diseases in veterinary orthopedics involve arthritis at some stage. Such common problems as cruciate ligament tears and hip dysplasia are ultimately diseases of osteoarthritis (OA) if left untreated. Developmental diseases, such as Legg-Perthes' disease and osteochondritis dessicans, have OA as a sequela. Forms of arthritis, such as immune-mediated disease, septic arthritis, and tick-borne arthritis, also become problems in veterinary practice. This article primarily reviews the pathophysiology, diagnosis, and therapy of OA but also briefly discusses immune-mediated arthritides.

PATHOPHYSIOLOGY OF OSTEOARTHRITIS

OA has been defined as "an inherently noninflammatory disorder of movable joints characterized by deterioration of articular cartilage and by the formation of new bone at the joint surfaces and margins" [1]. This syndrome, because of similar clinical signs (eg, pain, disability, swelling), must be differentiated from inflammatory arthritides. Although OA does have an inflammatory component, it is not characterized by the influx of inflammatory cells seen in the other joint diseases. In human beings, OA has been estimated to affect 85% of the population between ages 70 and 79 [2].

Because OA primarily affects the diarthrodial joints, a basic understanding of the anatomy and physiology of normal joint tissues is a prerequisite to further discussion. The typical diarthrodial joint is composed of two bones covered by articular cartilage and enclosed by a joint capsule that contains synovial fluid. Articular cartilage is the primary tissue involved in OA. The main function of normal articular cartilage is to provide a smooth, durable, low-friction joint surface and distribute load bearing from one bone to the other [2–4]. Cartilage

E-mail address: renberg@vet.k-state.edu

0195-5616/05/$ – see front matter
doi:10.1016/j.cvsm.2005.05.005

is an aneural and avascular tissue composed of chondrocytes imbedded in an acellular matrix. The chondrocytes are not surrounded by lacunae but are in intimate contact with the surrounding matrix [5].

Articular cartilage can be divided histologically into several zones, and the arrangement of chondrocytes gradually varies among these zones. The most superficial zone (farthest from the subchondral bone) is the tangential or gliding zone. In this layer the cells are flattened and elongated and are arranged parallel to the joint surface [5,6]. The large transitional zone lies deep to the first and contains cells that are more rounded and arranged in a random manner [5,6]. Below the transitional zone is the radial zone, in which cells are arrayed in columns perpendicular to the tidemark—an irregular line at the junction of the noncalcified and the calcified regions of the cartilage that stains blue with hematoxylin and eosin [5,6]. The precise function of the tidemark is not understood. Beneath the tidemark is the calcified zone, in which the cells are arranged in columns in a calcified matrix. The calcified zone is supported by the subchondral bone plate. The calcified cartilage joins the subchondral bone at the osteochondral junction. The undulating nature of the osteochondral junction is important for transmission of force from articular cartilage to bone.

Hyaline articular cartilage is approximately 70% to 80% water by weight [5]. This water is dispersed throughout the matrix, and its presence depends on the collagen and proteoglycan (PG) components of the matrix. The PG comprises approximately 35% of the matrix on a dry weight basis, and associated glycoproteins comprise an additional 10% [6]. The PG component of articular cartilage is found primarily in the transitional and radial zones. PG is produced in the golgi apparatus of chondrocytes and is composed of a core protein to which sidechains of glycosaminoglycan (GAG) molecules are covalently attached [7,8]. The classic description is that the PG core and its associated GAGs resemble a test tube brush. The GAGs have a distinct negative charge associated with sulfate groups at their free end, which results in the molecule being strongly hydrophilic [5,6]. Its negative charge also helps maintain the spatial structure of the cartilage under compressive loading. As a compressive load is applied to the articular cartilage, the noncompressible water resists the force. If the force is maintained, the water is gradually expelled from the matrix, which results in a pattern of visco-elastic deformation [4,8].

Most PG subunits in normal articular cartilage are bound by a link protein to hyaluronan [5]. Hyaluronan is a GAG that forms the backbone of a large (60–150 million d) molecule known as aggrecan [5]. There are four primary GAGs: chondroitin-4-sulfate, chondroitin-6-sulfate, keratan sulfate, and dermatan sulfate. The two forms of chondroitin sulfate are longer than the other two GAGs [5]. The GAG types are not arranged randomly on the protein core but are consistently found in particular domains at certain distances from the link protein. Alterations to this arrangement form the basis of identifying the changes that occur to PG in articular cartilage in osteoarthritic joints, namely, that the amount of the chondroitin sulfate increases relative to keratan sulfate [7]. In normal cartilage, it is possible to extract only a small amount of PG with various solvents, which indicates that the PG is firmly attached to the collagen network [7]. This situation contrasts with the situation in diseased joints, which suggests that the PG is being disrupted and is less tightly aggregated.

Another major component of the articular cartilage matrix is collagen. Collagen molecules are designed in triple helices that form fibrils and fibers, which serve to impart most of the tensile strength to the cartilage [2,4]. Type II collagen comprises as much as 90% of the total collagen in normal articular cartilage, but types I, III, V, VI, IX, X, and XI also may be present [5,6]. The collagen fibers are oriented uniquely in each zone of articular cartilage, and the orientation corresponds to the orientation of chondrocytes in that zone. For example, in the tangential zone, collagen fibrils are parallel to the joint surface; in the transitional zone they are obliquely arranged; and the fibrils are perpendicular to the surface and the tidemark in the radial zone [5].

Heterogeneity of the matrix is observed on the ultrastructural level with electron microscopy. The area immediately surrounding the chondrocytes, the pericellular matrix, contains a different GAG distribution than the matrix further from the chondrocyte. The pericellular matrix contains a higher percentage of chondroitin sulfate, whereas the interterritorial matrix, which is slightly further away, contains more keratan sulfate [9]. The distribution of collagen types also depends on location. Type VI collagen is found in the pericellular region and may serve to link the cells to larger collagen fibers [10].

Interactions between the various components of articular cartilage are complex and incompletely understood. The negative charge associated with the GAGs serves to maintain their spatial separation and contributes to the osmotic gradient. The osmotic pull attracts water into the matrix from the synovial fluid [6]. The amount of water imbibed is limited in part by the elastic limits imposed by the collagen fibers [8]. The water and the negative charge density give cartilage its ability to counter compression from load bearing by increasing turgor and evenly distributing the load. The load-bearing ability of cartilage is optimized by the damping effect of visco-elastic creep, whereby during prolonged load bearing the water is slowly exuded from the cartilage [6]. The water forced from the cartilage also contributes to joint lubrication [5]. When the load is released, water slowly returns to the cartilage, which aids in the diffusion of nutrients and the elimination of cellular waste products. This long-accepted role of the pumping mechanism in delivering nutrients to articular cartilage has been questioned [11].

In addition to articular cartilage, a diarthrodial joint is composed of joint capsule, synovial fluid, and subchondral bone. The joint capsule is composed of several layers. Its outer, thick, fibrous portion and surrounding connective tissue primarily fulfill a support role. The synovium, which is the inner layer, contains blood vessels and nerves and is important in maintaining the volume of synovial fluid. It is involved in various disease processes that affect joints. The synovium has no basement membrane and may be only a few cells thick in normal patients. Synoviocytes are classified as either type A, which are mainly phagocytic, or type B, which are mainly secretory. The synovial fluid itself is often called an ultrafiltrate of plasma because it is similar to plasma but does not contain many of the large molecules found in plasma. In addition to maintaining joint homeostasis, synovial fluid provides lubrication. The water that is forced out of the cartilage with compressive loads separates the opposing surfaces and provides a lubricating function, which is termed "weeping lubrication." When no compressive loads are being applied, the synovial fluid itself provides a lubricating role through the actions of substances such as hyaluronic acid and lubricin [6], which is termed boundary lubrication. Research has shown that the actual lubricant may be a surface active phospholipid, whereas lubricin acts as a carrier molecule [12].

The subchondral bone of the epiphysis is arranged in a lattice work configuration that allows for the transmission of forces of weight bearing from the articular cartilage cap to the cortex of the adjoining bones [13]. The cartilage is not connected structurally to the bone but interdigitates with subchondral bone at the osteochondral junction to provide a stable attachment [8]. This interdigitation allows shear forces to be converted to less destructive compressive forces. Subchondral bone is more pliable than cortical bone and can distribute the forces it absorbs more readily. In diseased joints, the subchondral bone may become thickened or sclerotic, which decreases its compliance and forces the cartilage to absorb more forces of weight bearing.

The pathophysiology of OA has been studied extensively but is still incompletely understood. The disease process itself involves several events that interact to form a self-perpetuating and progressively more severe cycle. In many cases, an inciting event is difficult to identify. In animals, unlike in humans, OA without evidence of underlying causes is rare. Normal joints do not undergo deterioration with normal forces; however, subjecting a normal joint may initiate OA [6,14]. In many researchers' opinion, the primary pathophysiologic event in the progression of OA is PG loss, but this is not the inciting change [8]. Most commonly, OA begins with a disruption of the surface layer of the articular cartilage, and this physical damage initiates biochemical alterations that result in degradation of joint tissues [8,13]. Some researchers believe that the initial damage is not at the surface but rather involves loosening of the collagen bonds [4,15]. Other work has pointed to the role of changes in subchondral bone density. Mechanical conditions that result in uneven load bearings, such as gross incongruity of the joint, result in concentration of loading to a particular part of the joint, which leads to abnormal wear [8].

Disruption of the surface cartilage can occur for various reasons. Regardless of the inciting event, this disruption initiates several changes. Surface disruption, which is termed fibrillation, resembles "flaking" on histologic evaluation because collagen fibers in this zone are arranged parallel to the joint surface [16]. Fibrillation initially causes disruption parallel to the collagen fibers, but with disease progression the disruption becomes perpendicular. When integrity of the cartilage is damaged, its ability to transmit and resist loads is diminished. Initially the mechanical functions of cartilage decrease because of increased water content secondary to loss of the restraining properties of collagen fibrils. Later they decrease because of general loss of matrix and the resulting cartilage thinning, which results in the initial fibrillation becoming fissures in the deeper layers of the cartilage. These physical disruptions may cause the collagen cross-linkages to break, which may in turn allow initial losses of PG [15]. Fibrillation also frees small fragments of cartilage matrix in the synovial fluid, where they are phagocitized by the synovium. This occurrence causes an inflammatory synovitis [17,18]. Some experimental work has suggested that PG fragments may be the component responsible for the inflammatory synovitits [19].

As fibrillation continues, chondrocyte damage occurs and more PG is lost. As the mechanical damage further degrades the weight-distributing function of the cartilage, the subchondral bone also is subjected to higher loads and responds by becoming more rigid and sclerotic and is less able to absorb and transfer forces from the cartilage to bone [15,20]. Without the protective mechanisms provided by a normal matrix, articular cartilage becomes more susceptible to further damage during normal weight bearing and a vicious cycle of disease progression is set in motion.

Gross changes of an osteoarthritic joint depend on the severity of the disease and, to some extent, the underlying cause. Initially, the joint capsule is thickened by fibrin and inflammatory edema secondary to the synovitis, and synovial villous hypertrophy may be present [5,21,22]. Effusion is often present and is likely the result of increased vascular permeability secondary to inflammation, increased proximity of synovial capillaries to the joint space secondary to capsule stretching, or increased osmotic gradient associated with the increased cellular and protein content of the synovial fluid [6]. The cartilage surface often displays a dull appearance and may be pebbled and rough [5]. As degenerative changes progress, fissures may be evident, and ultimately, areas of cartilage erosion develop. The exposed underlying bone often takes on a polished appearance known as eburnation. Severe changes are first seen in areas of the joint most subject to the stresses of load bearing (eg, the craniodorsal region in the canine hip) [5,23].

Bony changes from OA also occur in the trabecular portion of the medullary canal and in the region of joint capsule attachment [24]. When an affected bone is sectioned longitudinally, it is noted that the trabeculae are dense and irregular, the cortex may be thickened, and the subchondral bone plate may be sclerotic. At the point of joint capsule attachment and along the articular margin, bony proliferations known as enthesophytes and osteophytes, respectively, may develop. These proliferations become radiographically evident as they enlarge and ossify. The cause of this bony proliferation is not completely understood but may represent an inflammatory response of the synovium and perichondrium, perhaps in response to stretching or as an effect of vascular ingrowth into the cartilage in the area [6,20].

Histologic changes associated with OA are predictable based on the preceding discussion. Early changes include evidence of fibrillation of the cartilage and a decreased ability of the cartilage to take up metachromatic stains with a cationic charge, such as Safranin O or Alcian Blue [6,7]. The loss of metachromasia indicates loss of PG along with its characteristic anionic charge. As fibrillation becomes more severe, vertical fissures develop. Chondrocytes exhibit cloning, an essentially pathognomonic finding in OA [5]. As the disease progresses, osteophytes become evident at the periphery of the joint. Changes in the joint capsule vary. The subsynovium and synovium may be thickened or may be of normal cellularity. Both layers may show a marked inflammatory cell infiltrate [5]. Blood vessels may penetrate the tidemark, and in the more severe stages the cartilage may be completely absent in areas of high load bearing [6]. The trabecular portion of underlying bone may show evidence of new bone formation, and the subchondral region is often thickened and sclerotic [5,24,25].

Chondrocyte damage is significant in several ways. Despite the chondrocytes' ability to respond to and repair minor injury by increased anabolism, a point is reached at which they can no longer compensate [26]. As their ability to maintain homeostasis is compromised, they begin to produce abnormal varieties of collagen and PG. Type I collagen, which is less biomechanically effective than type II collagen in weight distribution, may be produced. Some evidence suggests that cross-linking provided by type IX collagen also may be broken down [6]. The total water content of osteoarthritic cartilage increases because of loss of restraining tensile strength of the collagen fibers, which reduces the ability of the tissue to maintain its biomechanical properties.

The PG produced in the osteoarthritic joint is less aggregated with shorter GAG sidechains. Despite increased synthesis of PG, there is a net decrease caused by continuing loss [19]. PG loss results from the direct effects of physical damage to cartilage and from the actions of various degradative enzymes released by diseased chondrocytes [8]. Increased water content results in increased diffusion of large molecules, such as PG, which contributes to their loss [6]. The actions of protease enzymes on PG include cleavage of the core protein and disruption of links to hyaluronic acid molecules [26], which results in shorter PG molecules.

The synovial cells in an osteoarthritic joint also play a role in disease progression [27]. That synovitis observed in arthritic joints can either precede or follow cartilage change implies several pathophysiologic mechanisms for degenerative joint disease [28]. This synovitis is likely secondary to exposure of neoantigens on the fragments or other proinflammatory sequences on the cartilage [21,29]. Synovitis caused by phagocytosis of cartilage fragments prompts release of various biochemical mediators [2,19]. These mediators, or cytokines, stimulate the production of proteases by chondrocytes [29]. Synovitis is seen as early as 1 to 8 weeks after injury in experimental models but is less pronounced by 13 weeks [18,27]. Histologic changes observed in the synovium include a mononuclear cell infiltrate within 1 week, synovial cell pleomorphism by 2 weeks, and synovial cell foamy cytoplasm and vacuolation. These changes are most prominent at 8 to 12 weeks in experimental OA [18,30]. Synovitis produced by arthrotomy can result in mild cartilage lesions consistent with early OA [15,31,32]. In general, however, the progressive lesions typical of natural and experimental arthritis seem to require some additional insult, such as joint instability [15,28,33].

As research on the pathophysiology of OA progresses, the importance of biochemical mediators and degradative enzymes has been established. Several enzymes are likely to play a role in the disease. The primary ones belong to three families: serine, cysteine, and metalloproteases. The metalloproteases may be the most important enzymes, especially those specific enzymes known as collagenase and stromelysin. Collagenase promotes the breakdown of collagen in the cartilage matrix, whereas stromelysen, along with acid proteases, primary affects the PG [34]. In contrast to rheumatoid arthritis (RA), in which the enzymes seem to arise primarily from the synoviocytes, with OA the chondrocytes produce most of these enzymes [26,34]. Protease production by chondrocytes is supported by the fact that collagen destruction is initially pericellular. Chondrocytes that produce proteases seem to be located more densely in outer layers of articular cartilage [29]. The amount of collagenase recovered from cartilage is proportional to the severity of lesions [29]. That the enzymes are produced by the chondrocytes themselves and do not simply diffuse from synovial cells or other sources was supported by further studies by Pelletier and colleagues [27] in which levels of the enzymes in the synovial membrane and in the cartilage did not correlate with each other.

Degradative enzymes are initially produced in an inactive form and must be activated. Plasmin plays a vital role in activation [29]. Plasmin is formed in the inactive form plasminogen and must be transformed by plasminogen activator. Similarly, stomelysin likely plays a role in activating procollagenase to collagenase [26].

Although the control of protease production is complex and is incompletely understood, part of its regulation seems to be via inhibitor substances. Tissue inhibitors of metalloproteases (TIMP) are the best known and exist in at least two forms (TIMP-1 and TIMP-2) [26,34]. Inhibitor substances interact with specific receptors, which are currently being identified and characterized. In OA, the relative amount of TIMP is decreased, and the enzymatic degradation of cartilage is allowed to progress. Plasminogen activator also has an inhibitor, which ultimately serves to decrease the amount of plasmin and likely modulates the production of various cytokines and enzymes [34]. Plasminogen activator itself may have a direct degradative effect [35].

Biochemical mediators, called cytokines, are vital at the most basic level of the disease process. In normal joints, cytokines are integral in maintaining normal cartilage homeostasis. Among the cytokines, interleukin-1 (IL-1), IL-6, and tumor necrosis factor-α have been studied most extensively. In the diseased joint, these mediators are believed to be released primarily by inflamed synoviocytes, chondrocytes, and monocytes [19,26,34]. IL-1 specifically has an inhibitory effect on TIMP and indirectly promotes the degradative role of the metalloproteases [2]. IL-1 likely also decreases the chondrocytes' synthesis of collagen and PG while increasing the production PGE_2 [26,34].

IL-1 also activates macrophages and serves to stimulate the production of other inflammatory mediators and degradative enzymes by chondrocytes and synovial cells [6]. These individual actions of IL-1 may occur by completely different pathways, which complicates approaches to therapy.

Tumor necrosis factor-α produces various effects, many of which are similar to IL-1. It has direct and indirect catabolic effects on cartilage and may serve to activate IL-6. IL-6, in turn, is less well understood. Although it seems to decrease cartilage matrix synthesis, particularly PG, it also may stimulate TIMP. Additionally, IL-6 may promote the formation of chondrocyte clones [26]. Currently, control and regulation of cytokine production are only poorly understood.

Other mediators of inflammation that are of varying degrees of importance in the pathophysiology of arthritis exist. For example, the coagulation, kinin, and complement systems all play roles in the disease [2]. Activation of the coagulation cascade leads to the deposition of fibrin. Fibrin also may be produced in response to IL-1 and seems to be chemotactic for neutrophils. Neutrophils, in turn, release elastase and cathepsin-G, which degrade cartilage. Activation of the kinin system also may occur with activation of the coagulation cascade; bradykinin is a mediator of pain and may cause bone erosion [2].

In addition to these plasma-derived systems, inflammatory mediators also arise from cell membrane-associated systems. Phospholipases can act on the cell membrane to cause activation of the cyclo-oxygenase and lipoxygenase cascades. The resulting prostaglandins and leukotrienes serve chemotactic and vasoactive roles and are involved as mediators of pain. Prostaglandins, such as PGE_2, are found in increased concentrations in affected joints [2].

The overall result of the combined effects of PG loss, chondrocyte damage, collagen changes, and activity of biochemical mediators is that the cartilage is weaker and less able to function normally. This results in further physical damage to the cartilage and initiates a vicious cycle of painful arthritic disease.

DIAGNOSIS OF OSTEOARTHRITIS

The diagnosis of OA is typically not a difficult one and can be supported by physical examination findings, cytology, or imaging. The signs of arthritis found on physical examination include pain upon manipulation of the joint, periarticlar swelling, palpable effusion, and crepitis. These signs are somewhat nonspecific and must be combined with further diagnostics, compatible history, and clinical judgment. The history may include incidences of injuries or prior disease states, or the patient may be of a breed predisposed to OA-related problems. The signs of OA on radiographs vary with the severity of the disease but include effusion, osteophytosis, and subchondral sclerosis. Joint collapse may be evident on standing (weight bearing) films but is inconsistent and unreliable in small animals. Many investigators have studied the possibility of using biochemical markers to diagnosis arthritis before clinical signs develop or to predict the progression of the disease. Such work continues to be fraught with complications and variabilities that have limited its clinical usefulness to date [36,37].

The job of the clinician in diagnosing OA is not so much one of being alert to the possibility or likelihood of the disease but more one of eliminating alternative or additional possibilities. Many animals have OA in one or more joints, particularly as they age. Determining if the OA is the source of the clinical problem occasionally can be difficult. For example, a large-breed dog may have evidence of OA in its hips because of dysplasia, but the signs observed by the owners could be more related to lumbosacral disease that is not evident on radiographs. The most important aid in eliminating the chance of other problems is a thorough physical examination [38]. Ultimately it is up to the clinician to decide which of the clinical findings are significant and which are most related to the primary problem.

Sometimes the presence of arthritic change is obvious and is clearly the source of the patient's trouble. The arthritis may not be merely OA, however, and may require different management. Immune-mediated arthritis or infectious arthritis must be eliminated (or confirmed) before appropriate treatment can be initiated. History and signalment may be sufficient to make a diagnosis. Further diagnostic steps revolve around cytologic evaluation of the joint fluid, specifically the number of nucleated cells and their type. A simple method of thinking about joint fluid interpretation is to consider OA as having moderate elevations in cell counts, whereas the inflammatory arthritides have high counts. Normal joint fluid should have nucleated cell counts of approximately 300 to 500 cells/mL. Animals that suffer from OA typically have elevated counts, but the numbers are less than 5000 cells/mL [39]. OA is classified as a "noninflammatory" arthritis because of the cells found in the joint fluid. Animals with OA should have primarily mononuclear cell populations in the fluid. In contrast, the inflammatory arthritides have primarily a polymorphonuclear cell population. The further diagnostic evaluation of inflammatory arthritis is discussed later.

MANAGEMENT OF OSTEOARTHRITIS

Management of OA can be either surgical or conservative. Surgical management typically involves addressing the primary cause or performing salvage procedures. There are three main components to conservative management of OA: weight control, exercise/physical therapy, and medication. The precise protocols vary with the preferences of the clinician, the needs of the animal, and the abilities or desires of the owner.

Surgical options to address the primary problem are most effective in the early stages of the disease process. For example, addressing a torn cranial cruciate ligament via surgical intervention helps to alleviate pain and decreases the progression of arthritis. If the problem is longstanding, however, significant OA already will be present in the joint and the patient still will have signs consistent with the OA. In addition to torn ligaments, conditions such as osteochondrosis, hip dysplasia, elbow dysplasia, articular fractures, and growth deformities may be treated effectively through surgery to reduce or eliminate arthritic advancement.

Surgery is also helpful in alleviating the signs of arthritis when salvage procedures are performed. A salvage procedure is one that eliminates the joint (or limb) in an effort to alleviate the signs associated with the joint disease. Such procedures may be as simple as femoral head and neck ostectomies or as complex as joint replacement or arthrodesis. The outcomes after these surgeries may vary, and they generally can be performed at any time during the course of the OA. For this reason, most surgeons advocate performing salvage procedures only after conservative management has failed.

Conservative management is familiar at least in part to most owners. The use of medication to alleviate the symptoms of OA in the human population is widespread. Despite this familiarity, owners need extensive education in the appropriate management strategy for an individual patient. One of the most basic components of conservative management is weight control. Significant reductions in clinical signs can be seen when overweight dogs with OA lose weight. Although the animals should not be made excessively thin, the less weight a joint supports, the less deterioration it undergoes, all else being equal. Careful discussion of weight loss is critical, and guidelines can be found in many textbooks.

Exercise control and physical therapy are also vital to the management of OA. In the most general sense, the goals are to maintain joint mobility and muscle strength while minimizing additional joint destruction or pain. In this sense, exercise is an important benefit to the patient that has arthritis [40–42]. The optimal amount of exercise for a patient that has arthritis varies with the individual and with the stage of disease. Owners often desire a defined protocol immediately upon diagnosis, but unfortunately that is not possible. The veterinarian instead must convey the goals of activity and communicate ways to achieve them and what to watch for. One starting point is to compare the amount of activity the patient currently receives with the severity of the clinical signs and the fitness or body condition of the animal. Owners of relatively inactive animals with minimal signs should be encouraged to increase the pet's activity. This increase should be done gradually and in a controlled manner. It may be helpful to draw analogies to a person who is out of shape but decides to take up running. The owners should monitor the pet's clinical signs after exercise and the next day. If the patient seems less comfortable, then the exercise should be decreased in duration, frequency, or intensity. The exercise regimen and the monitoring of clinical signs should be done while considering any medical management that is occurring. Changes in one factor affect the need and use of the other. Clients should be instructed to look for willingness to continue play and exercise, ability to climb stairs or enter vehicles, general activity, comfort during other physical therapy, and changes in lameness.

At the other end of the spectrum from the inactive patient with minimal signs is the animal that suffers significantly from OA while maintaining an active lifestyle (voluntarily or involuntarily). Some animals have such a desire for play that they constantly pursue activity despite discomfort and worsening of their signs afterwards. Other animals may perform tasks or roles obediently because they have been asked to do so. Owners with animals that show evidence of discomfort from OA should back off on the animals' allowed activity until significant improvement in signs is noted. Activity then can be increased gradually in an effort to find a level that does not exacerbate the signs. Play time or work activities may be divided effectively into more numerous episodes of shorter duration or lower intensity in an effort to not deprive the animal of its primary function or enjoyment. Although excessive weight loss can be detrimental to an animal's health, strong correlation can be found between supranormal body weight and lameness [43].

A discussion of physical therapy is beyond the scope of this article, but veterinarians should be aware of the importance of such intervention for patients that have arthritis. Treatments as simple as passive range-of-motion exercises by owners may provide significant relief. Similarly, owners easily can provide massage, heat or cold therapy, and even aquatherapy if they receive instruction. These modalities and more are offered increasingly by trained veterinarians or veterinary technicians, but many owners with chronically affected pets are unable to continue such sessions. For this reason, home therapy is frequently the best option.

The last component of conservative management is the use of medications, such as nonsteroidal anti-inflammatory drugs (NSAIDs), slow-acting, disease-modifying OA agents (eg, neutraceuticals or chondroprotectives), and intra-articular agents. The use of these agents is complicated, and concrete guidelines are almost impossible to draw from the current literature. A brief overview of their use is provided in this article.

The foundation of medical management is the use of NSAIDs. Many different products are available on the veterinary market, and new drugs are released every year as research into this area continues. The various drugs are grouped because of their anti-inflammatory actions via interruption of portions of the arachidonic acid cascade. Chiefly, the drugs work by inhibiting cyclo-oxygenase. More and more, the use of cyclo-oygenase-2 preferential drugs has become possible and preferable. These drugs tend to have less risk of gastrointestinal side effects, but much is still unknown about their mechanism and use. They likely have similar efficacy as traditional NSAIDs [44].

NSAIDs are effective and generally safe, but they must be used carefully. The possibility of gastrointestinal, renal, hepatic, and other side effects is real. In general, the use of appropriate doses in animals without predisposing conditions and under supervision by the owners is without trouble. Because many of the patients with OA are older (and may be more likely to have concurrent disease) and will be given the drugs for a prolonged time, frequent assessment is important. If signs develop, the drugs should be stopped and the animal should undergo observation for a period of time (up to several weeks) before trying a different NSAID. Avoiding human products is mandatory. In dogs, as in humans, the use of acetaminophen may be a valuable alternative or supplement to NSAIDs. Acetaminophen generally is found to be less effective but safer than the NSAIDs [45]. Tramadol, a dual mechanism analgesic, is being used in veterinary medicine, although little is known about its safety or pharmacokinetics [46].

The manufacturer's recommended dose should be viewed as a starting point. Many animals can achieve relief on lesser doses or less frequent dosing. Some animals may require medication only in the time period surrounding increased activity (eg, weekends or hunting season). Just as with exercise, clinicians must work with clients closely to determine the lowest effective dose and monitor for complications. Some animals may have such severity of signs that NSAIDs alone are ineffective at controlling the pain.

The use of corticosteroids in the treatment of OA remains controversial. Although these agents reduce synovitis and inflammatory changes in the cartilage, they also may be detrimental to cartilage health by decreasing PG and collagen production [47]. The intra-articular use of corticosteroids may lessen systemic side effects, but their use has been associated with a steroid arthropathy. Several different long-acting steroids have been used intra-articularly, and the differences are incompletely understood. Given the controversy concerning the balance between detrimental and therapeutic effects, the author considers intra-articular use of corticosteroids to be a valid option in the short-term but a poor long-term solution.

Long-term therapy in many cases involves the use of slow-acting, disease-modifying OA agents, such as glucosamine and hyaluronan. These agents have sometimes been termed neutraceuticals or chondroprotective agents, depending on their formulation and perceived mode of action. Anecdotal evidence abounds to support the use of such therapies, but a healthy skepticism exists because of the dearth of well-controlled prospective trials. Oral products have received a great deal of publicity. Therapeutic benefit to these drugs is supported by some studies and may be caused by either anti-inflammatory activity (more properly, antireactive activity because the effect is likely independent of the arachidonic acid cascade) [48] or supplying the components and cofactors necessary for cartilage repair [47]. Glucosamine is available in several forms, including glucosamine hydrochloride, glucosamine sulfate, and N-acetyl-glucosamine. Most studies have been performed on the sulfate version, although it is unclear whether some forms are more effective than others (potentially the N-acetyl version is less efficacious) [49,50]. One should remember that despite positive reports, other studies show no benefit from these products [51]. A similar product, pentosan polysulfate, is not available in the United States but has shown promise in various trials elsewhere [52]. Some investigations have pointed to the value of omega-6/omega-3 balance or supplementation in treating arthritis [53]. The general premise is that certain fatty acids (primarily omega-3) may be able to compete with others for incorporation and conversion of inflammatory mediators from arachidonic acid [49]. The prostaglandins and leukotrienes derived from omega-3 fatty acids are generally noninflammatory. Several diets that are currently available have shown clinical promise in combating the symptoms of OA.

Other slow-acting, disease-modifying OA agents include injectable products, such as polysulfated GAG. These drugs show promise in decreasing direct and indirect evidence of OA in vitro, but clinical studies are more equivocal [47,54,55]. Hyaluronan also has been used intra-articularly with similarly confusing results. It may have efficacy related to increasing viscosity and an anti-inflammatory action. One meta-analysis revealed a generally high level of safety and reliable efficacy, although the degree of improvement varied and heterogeneity between studies limited the conclusions [56]. There is no consensus as to the importance of the variation in molecular weight of the various formulations [57]. Intra-articular treatments in small animal practice are not common but are used relatively frequently in human medicine [58–60]. Corticosteroids and hyaluronan have some efficacy, with steroids providing faster relief of shorter duration.

Based on the various options available for medical management of OA and the lack of clarity as to efficacy and optimal protocols, veterinary clinicians may be excused for finding some freedom in choosing treatment regimens. Clinicians also should note a deep responsibility to remain abreast of new developments and recommendations. There is no current way to predict reliably which treatments, especially with regard to slow-acting, disease-modifying OA agents, will be best for an individual patient [49]. New drugs are constantly being developed, and new uses for current drugs, such as bisphosphonates or free radical scavengers, may be of benefit in the treatment of OA [49,61]. Severe cases of OA in veterinary patients, as in humans, likely would benefit from combination therapy (eg, use acetaminophen, opioids, or slow-acting, disease-modifying OA agents in additional to traditional NSAIDs) [62]. Few, if any, investigations have studied such therapy in veterinary medicine.

RHEUMATOID ARTHRITIS

In addition to OA, veterinary patients may suffer from immune-mediated arthritides. These diseases are typically considered based on presentation and joint fluid analysis. Patients may present with varying degrees of lameness but usually have a polyarthropathy of the more distal joints. An animal with multiple joint pain always should be suspected of having a polyarthropathy, and arthrocentesis should be performed. Radiographs may be performed to determine better the extent and severity of the disease and check for erosive lesions, but they are not always helpful in influencing treatment. The immune-mediated arthritides have been classified as erosive or nonerosive, and this classification may help determine the specific disease. Clinically, a definitive diagnosis beyond that of immune-mediated arthritis is not always necessary.

None of the immune-mediated arthritides is common in animals, but RA may occur more frequently than others. RA is a significant disease in the human population and has been studied extensively. Despite this, it is still poorly understood. Simplistically, RA occurs when a patient's immune system forms autoantibodies against IgG. These antibodies, termed RF for rheumatoid factor, form complexes with the IgG [63,64]. The complexes become deposited in the synovium and create an inflammatory response. The response is primarily humoral in nature, with less involvement from T cells [65,66]. The aggressive inflammation leads to severe destruction of the cartilage and other joint tissues, including loss of the underlying bone.

The underlying cause for the development of RF against the host IgG remains unknown. The initiating event may be a change in the native IgG that renders it antigenic or there may be a defect in the body's ability to maintain self-tolerance [67]. Some researchers have suggested that the RF may have some degree of physiologic function, as reported by Dorner and colleagues [65]. Possibly the magnitude of the response to the RF separates the RA patient, not the presence of the RF alone. These thoughts are supported by the observation that RF may be present in various disease processes, but its presence is usually transient and not directly detrimental [65]. Of additional interest, some correlation between the presence of canine distemper virus titers and RA has never been fully explained and may yet yield some insight into the pathogenesis of the disease [68,69]. In veterinary medicine, the disease is found predominantly in small or toy breeds, with no gender predilection [67]. Shetland sheepdogs may be overrepresented [70].

Various laboratory tests assist in the diagnosis of RA. The primary test is cytologic evaluation of the joint fluid, which should yield a predominantly neutrophilic population with significantly elevated cell counts (approximately 50,000). Additional tests include checking antinuclear antibody and RF, but both tests have equivocal results. In general, a positive RF test result supports the diagnosis, but it may not be highly specific. One study supported the use of a more specific test for IgA-RF as opposed to IgM-RF, but the assays may not be widely available [71]. As with OA, substantial research is being conducted into the search for synovial markers of disease. One interesting study noted a dramatic increase in metalloproteases, such as MMP-3, that is poorly balanced by TIMP. This is in contrast to OA findings and could be a useful diagnostic aid [72]. In the human field, well-defined criteria characterize RA, and a certain number must be fulfilled to have a positive diagnosis. Although some of the criteria transfer to the canine patient, the use of the list is less helpful—and less critical—for veterinary patients in this author's opinion. Once a diagnosis of immune-mediated arthritis is made, a suspicion of RA can be bolstered by noting the presence of erosive lesions on radiographs. RA, much like erosive polyarthritis of greyhounds and feline chronic progressive polyarthritis, elicits activation of osteoclasts, in contrast to the other immune-mediated arthritides. Subsequent repair efforts result in substantial joint fibrosis or subluxation [67].

Treatment of RA is similar to the treatment for other immune-mediated diseases, namely, the use of immunosuppressive drugs (sometimes called disease-modifying, antirheumatic drugs). Although prednisone has been the mainstay of therapy, many clinicians find the need to use a combination of drugs, such as azathioprine, cyclophosphamide, or methotrexate or even gold salts [63,73,74]. There is currently no curative treatment for RA, so the treatment goals center on remission of clinical signs and return to reasonable function. The use of NSAIDs may be of value in some cases, but their use in patients that are also receiving steroids or other disease-modifying, antirheumatic drugs is contraindicated. Because of the greater efficacy of the latter drugs, NSAIDs are used less often in the treatment of veterinary patients that have RA. General guidelines for initial therapy of RA with prednisone can be found in many texts [67,73,75]. Because of the aggressive nature of the disease, some clinicians recommend early therapy with other immunosuppressive drugs either in addition to the prednisone or alone. Such therapy may involve the use of various agents, but azathioprine and cyclophosphamide are probably the most common. Methotrexate has been advocated in the treatment of humans who have RA, but the author is unaware of documented use in veterinary RA cases [74]. There are agents that more specifically target the actions of tumor necrosis factor or interleukins. These agents are not approved for veterinary use but may see application as experience increases.

Regardless of the specific drug protocol initially selected, early diagnosis is essential. Once substantial joint damage has occurred, even considerable success in halting progression will not restore function. Another key to practical success is the establishment of realistic expectations on the part of the owners. Remission of clinical signs likely may be only partial and temporary. Some type of therapy is needed for the duration of the animal's life. Finally, the comments concerning physical therapy, exercise, and weight control previously mentioned in regard to OA also apply to the immune-mediated arthropathies.

SYSTEMIC LUPUS ERYTHEMATOSUS

Another major immune-mediated arthropathy in veterinary medicine is systemic lupus erythematosus (SLE). SLE is a systemic disease with arthritic manifestations as the most common component [63]. The pathophysiology of SLE centers on the deposition of immune complexes. These complexes then incite inflammation wherever they are deposited. The resulting pathology can include glomerulonephritis, dermatitis, anemia, and thrombocytopenia, among other problems. The initiating cause of the complexes is unknown, with genetic, environmental, and transmissible factors suggested [76].

As with RA, diagnosis of SLE can be problematic because no one test or combination of tests easily yields a definitive diagnosis [76]. A positive antinuclear antibody test is helpful but is not specific. It is reasonably sensitive [76]. A positive test result for lupus erythematosus cell preparation is helpful but can be difficult. Lupus erythematosus cells are neutrophils that have phagocytized opsonized nuclear material. A positive result is considered relatively specific by some but may have questionable sensitivity because the concentration of such cells varies [63,64]. If a positive antinuclear antibody test result is found in conjunction with a positive LE cell test result, the differential of RA likely can be ruled out [77]. Ultimately, the diagnosis of SLE is made by noting the consistent clinical signs and finding some supportive laboratory data, including joint fluid analysis. As with RA, lists of clinical signs extrapolated from the human field may be used to support a diagnosis of SLE. Disagreement exists about the usefulness of these lists [76].

The treatment of SLE in dogs generally mirrors that of RA and revolves around immunosuppressive therapy. In addition to seeking symptomatic relief to the arthritis, clinicians must respond to failure or disease in any other organs involved. In general, the prognosis is poor because relapses are common. Reports on long-term survival vary widely [76].

Given the frequency of occurrence of arthritis in veterinary patients, it is crucial that clinicians be aware of the mechanisms of the disease and be comfortable with diagnosis and treatment. Unfortunately, there is a great deal of information still to be learned in regard to management of these cases. Because of the rapid and continuing research gains, it behooves clinicians to maintain a current awareness of the related literature.

References

[1] Hough A. Pathology of osteoarthritis. In: Koopman W, editor. Arthritis and allied conditions. 13th edition. Baltimore: Williams and Wilkins; 1997. p. 1945–68.

[2] Pettipher E. Pathogenesis and treatment of chronic arthritis. Sci Prog 1989;73:521–34.

[3] Morgan S. The pathology of canine hip dysplasia. Vet Clin North Am 1992;22:541–50.

[4] Mow V. Structure-function relationships of articular cartilage and the effects of joint instability and trauma on cartilage function. In: Brandt K, editor. Cartilage changes in osteoarthritis. Indianapolis (IN): Indiana University School of Medicine; 1990. p. 22–42.

[5] Mankin H. Normal articular cartilage and the alterations in osteoarthritis. In: Lombardino JG, editor. Nonsteroidal antiinflammatory drugs. New York: John Wiley and Sons; 1985. p. 1–73.

[6] Todhunter R. Synovial joint anatomy, biology, and pathobiology. In: Auer J, editor. Equine surgery. Philadelphia: WB Saunders; 1992. p. 844–65.

[7] Adams M, Billingham M. Animal models for degenerative joint disease. In: Berry CL, editor. Current topics in pathology, bone and joint disease. New York: Springer-Verlag; 1982. p. 521–34.

[8] Teitelbaum S, Bullough P. The pathophysiology of bone and joint disease. Am J Pathol 1979;96:283–354.

[9] Poole C. The structure and function of articular cartilage matrices. In: Woessner J, Howell D, editors. Joint cartilage degradation. New York: Marcel Dekker, Inc.; 1993. p. 1–36.

[10] Mayne R, Brewton R. Extracellular matrix of cartilage: collagen. In: Woessner J, Howell D, editors. Joint cartilage degradation. New York: Marcel Dekker, Inc.; 1993. p. 81–108.

[11] Maroudas A, Bullough P, Swanson S. The permeability of articular cartilage. J Bone Joint Surg Br 1968;50B:166–77.

[12] Hills B. Remarkable anti-wear properties of joint surfactant. Ann Biomed Eng 1995;23:112–5.

[13] Radin E, Paul I, Lowy M. A comparison of the dynamic force transmitting properties of subchondral bone and articular cartilage. J Bone Joint Surg Am 1970;52A:444–56.

[14] Palmoski M, Brandt K. Running inhibits the reversal of atrophic changes in canine knee cartilage after removal of a leg cast. Arthritis Rheum 1981;24:1329–37.

[15] Burr D. Trauma as a factor in the initiation of osteoarthritis. In: Brandt K, editor. Cartilage changes in osteoarthritis. Indianapolis (IN): Indiana University School of Medicine; 1990. p. 63–72.

[16] Greisen H, Summers B, Lust G. Ultrastructure of the articular cartilage and synovium in the early stages of degenerative joint disease in canine hip joints. Am J Vet Res 1982;43:1963–71.

[17] Ghosh P, Smith M. The role of cartilage-derived antigens, pro-coagulant activity and fibrinolysis in the pathogenesis of osteoarthritis. Med Hypotheses 1993;41:190–4.

[18] Lipowitz A. Synovial membrane changes after experimental transection of the cranial cruciate ligament in dogs. Am J Vet Res 1985;46:1166–70.

[19] Boniface R, Cain P, Evans C. Articular responses to purified cartilage proteoglycans. Arthritis Rheum 1988;31:258–66.

[20] Alexander J. The pathogenesis of canine hip dysplasia. Vet Clin North Am 1992;22:503–11.

[21] Lust G, Summers B. Early, asymptomatic stage of degenerative joint disease in canine hip joints. Am J Vet Res 1981;42:1849–55.

[22] Myers S, Brandt K, Connor B, et al. Synovitis and osteoarthritic changes in canine articular cartilage after anterior cruciate ligament transection. Arthritis Rheum 1990;1990:1406–15.

[23] Riser W. The dysplastic hip joint: radiologic and histologic development. Vet Pathol 1975;12:279–305.

[24] Dedrick D, Goldstein S, Brandt K. A longitudinal study of subchondral plate and trabecular bone in cruciate-deficient dogs with osteoarthritis followed up for 54 months. Arthritis Rheum 1993;36:1460–7.

[25] Strom H, Svalastoga E. A quantitative assessment of the subchondral changes in osteoarthritis and its association to the cartilage degeneration. Veterinary Comparative Orthopaedics and Traumatology 1993;6:198–201.

[26] Pelletier J-P, DiBattista JA. Cytokines and inflammation in cartilage degradation. Rheum Dis Clin North Am 1993;19:545–68.

[27] Pelletier J-P, Martel-Pelletier J, Ghandur-Mnaymneh L, et al. Role of synovial membrane inflammation in cartilage matrix breakdown in the Pond-Nuki dog model of osteoarthritis. Arthritis Rheum 1985;28:554–61.

[28] Lukoschek M, Boyd R, Schaffler M, et al. Comparison of joint degeneration models. Acta Orthop Scand 1986;57:349–53.

[29] Pelletier J-P, Martel-Pelletier J. The pathophysiology of osteoarthritis and the implication of the use of hyaluronan and hylan as therapeutic agents in viscosupplementation. J Rheumatol 1993;20(Suppl):19–24.

[30] McDevit C, Gilbertson E, Muir H. An experimental model of osteoarthritis: early morphological and biochemical changes. J Bone Joint Surg Br 1977;59B:24–35.

[31] Lukoschek M, Schaffler M, Burr D. Synovial membrane and cartilage changes in experimental osteoarthrosis. J Orthop Res 1988;6:475–92.

[32] Pelletier J-P, Martel-Pelletier J, Altman R, et al. Collagenolytic activity and collagen matrix breakdown of the articular cartilage in the Pond-Nuki dog model of osteoarthritis. Arthritis Rheum 1983;26:866–74.

[33] Wigren A, Wik O, Falk J. Intra-articular injection of high-molecular hyaluronic acid. Acta Orthop Scand 1976;47:480–5.

[34] Pelletier J-P, Roughley P, DiBattista J. Are cytokines involved in osteoarthritic pathophysiology? Semin Arthritis Rheum 1991;20:12–25.

[35] Quigley J. Phorbol ester-induced morphological changes in transformed chick fibroblasts: evidence for direct catalytic involvement of plasminogen activator. Cell 1979;17:131–41.

[36] Garnero P, Delmas P. Biomarkers in osteoarthritis. Curr Opin Rheumatol 2003;15:641–6.

[37] Roughley P, El-Maadawy S. The use of biochemical markers of bone and cartilage metabolism to monitor osteoarthritis: dreams and reality. J Rheumatol 2003;30:910–2.

[38] Renberg W. Evaluation of the lame patient. Vet Clin North Am 2001;31:1–16.

[39] Ellison R. The cytologic examination of synovial fluid. Semin Vet Med Surg (Small Anim) 1988;3:133–9.

[40] Baar MV, Assendelft WJJ, Dekker J, et al. Effectiveness of exercise therapy in patients with osteoarthritis of the hip or knee. Arthritis Rheum 1999;42:1361–9.

[41] Millis D, Levine D. The role of exercise and physical modalities in the treatment of osteoarthritis. Vet Clin North Am Small Anim Pract 1997;27:913–29.

[42] Minor M. Impact of exercise on osteoarthritis outcomes. J Rheumatol 2004;31:81–6.

[43] Impellizeri J, Tetrick M, Muir P. Effect of weight reduction on clinical signs of lameness in dogs with hip osteoarthritis. JAVMA 2000;216:1089–91.

[44] Hochberg M. New directions in symptomatic therapy for patients with osteoarthritis and rheumatoid arthritis. Semin Arthritis Rheum 2002;32:4–14.

[45] Zhang W, Jones A, Doherty M. Does paracetamol (acetaminophen) reduce the pain of osteoarthritis? A meta-analysis of randomised controlled trials. Ann Rheum Dis 2004;63:901–7.

[46] Parker R. Tramadol. Compendium on Continuing Education for the Practicing Veterinarian 2004;26:800–2.

[47] Todhunter R, Johnston S. Osteoarthritis. In: Slatter D, editor. Textbook of small animal surgery. 3rd edition. Philadelphia: WB Saunders; 2003. p. 2208–46.

[48] Matheson A, Perry C. Glucosamine: a review of its use in the management of osteoarthritis. Drugs Aging 2003;20:1041–60.

[49] Beale B. Use of nutraceuticals and chondroprotectants in osteoarthritic dogs and cats. Vet Clin North Am 2004;34:271–89.

[50] Zerkak D, Dougados M. The use of glucosamine therapy in osteoarthritis. Curr Rheumatol Rep 2004;6:41–5.

[51] Cibere J, Kopec JA, Thorne A, et al. Randomized, double-blind, placebo-controlled glucosamine discontinuation trial in knee osteoarthritis. Arthritis Rheum 2004;51:738–45.

[52] Ghosh P. The pathobiology of osteoarthritis and the rationale for the use of pentosan polysulfate for its treatment. Semin Arthritis Rheum 1999;28:211–67.

[53] Cleland L, James M, Proudman S. Omega-6/Omega-3 fatty acids and arthritis. World Rev Nutr Diet 2003;92:152–68.

[54] Richette P, Bardin T. Structure-modifying agents for osteoarthritis: an update. Joint Bone Spine 2004;71:18–23.

[55] Todhunter R, Lust G. Polysulfated glycosaminoglycan in the treatment of osteoarthritis. JAVMA 1994;204:1245–51.

[56] Wang C-T, Lin J, Chang C-J, et al. Therapeutic effects of hyaluronic acid on osteoarthritis of the knee. J Bone Joint Surg Am 2004;86A:538–45.

[57] Kelly M, Moskowitz R, Lieberman J. Hyaluronan therapy: looking toward the future. Am J Orthop 2004;33(Suppl 1):23–8.

[58] Chard J, Dieppe P. Update: treatment of osteoarthritis. Arthritis Rheum 2002;47:686–90.

[59] Gossec L, Dougados M. Intra-articular treatments in osteoarthritis: from the symptomatic to the structure modifying. Ann Rheum Dis 2003;63:478–82.

[60] Uthman I, Raynould J-P, Haraoui B. Intra-articular therapy in osteoarthritis. Postgrad Med J 2003;79:449–53.

[61] Cohen S. An update on bisphosphonates. Curr Rheumatol Rep 2004;6:59–65.

[62] Altman R. Pain relief in osteoarthritis: the rationale for combination therapy. J Rheumatol 2004;31:5–7.

[63] Brunner C. Autoimmunity. In: Bonagura J, editor. Kirk's current veterinary therapy. 12th edition. Philadelphia: WB Saunders; 1995. p. 554–60.

[64] Shrader S. The use of the laboratory in the diagnosis of joint disorders of dogs and cats. In: Bonagura J, editor. Kirk's current veterinary therapy. 12th edition. Philadelphia: WB Saunders; 1995. p. 1166–70.

[65] Dorner T, Egerer K, Feist E, et al. Rheumatoid factor revisited. Curr Opin Rheumatol 2004;16:246–53.

[66] Vervoordeldonk M, Tak P. Cytokines in rheumatoid arthritis. Curr Rheumatol Rep 2002;4:208–17.

[67] Lewis R. Rheumatoid arthritis. Vet Clin North Am 1994;24:697–701.

[68] Bell S, Carter S, Bennett D. Canine distemper viral antigens and antibodies in dogs with rheumatoid arthritis. Res Vet Sci 1991;50:64–8.

[69] Carter S, Barnes A, Gilmore W. Canine rheumatoid arthritis and inflammatory cytokines. Vet Immunol Immunopathol 1999;69:201–14.

[70] Newton C, Lipowitz A. Canine rheumatoid arthritis: a brief review. J Am Anim Hosp Assoc 1975;11:595–9.

[71] Bell S, Carter S, May C, et al. IgA and IgM rheumatoid factors in canine rheumatoid arthritis. J Small Anim Pract 1993;34:259–64.

[72] Hegemann N, Wondimu A, Ullrich K, et al. Synovial MMP-3 and TIMP-1 levels and their correlation with cytokine expression in canine rheumatoid arthritis. Vet Immunol Immunopathol 2003;91:199–204.

[73] Bennett D. Treatment of the immune-based inflammatory arthropathies of the dog and cat. In: Bonagura J, editor. Kirk's current veterinary therapy. 12th edition. Philadelphia: WB Saunders; 1996. p. 1188–95.

[74] O'Dell J. Therapeutic strategies for rheumatoid arthritis. N Engl J Med 2004;350:2591–602.

[75] Davidson A. Immune-mediated polyarthritis. In: Slatter D, editor. Textbook of small animal surgery. Philadelphia: WB Saunders; 2003. p. 2246–50.

[76] Marks S, Henry C. CVT update: diagnosis and treatment of systemic lupus erythematosus. In: Bonagura J, editor. Kirk's current veterinary therapy. 13th edition. Philadelphia: WB Saunders; 2000. p. 514–6.

[77] Lipowitz A, Newton C. Laboratory parameter of rheumatoid arthritis of the dog: a review. J Am Anim Hosp Assoc 1975;11:600–6.

Vet Clin Small Anim 35 (2005) 1093–1109

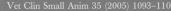

VETERINARY CLINICS
SMALL ANIMAL PRACTICE

Infections of the Skeletal System

Loretta J. Bubenik, DVM, MS

Companion Animal Surgery, Veterinary Clinical Sciences, Louisiana State University School
of Veterinary Medicine, Baton Rouge, LA 70803, USA

Osteomyelitis is defined as bone inflammation, but use of the term usually denotes bone infection. Septic arthritis refers to active joint infection, usually bacterial in origin. A variety of contributing factors play a role in bone and joint infections, but open fracture repair and joint penetration are frequent sources. Treatment and outcome vary depending on the source of infection, organism involved, and duration of infection.

MICROBIOLOGY

A variety of organisms contribute to orthopedic infection. For bone infections, a single organism is usually involved [1]. Multiple organisms are isolated 33% to 66% of the time [2–4]. β-Lactamase–producing staphylococcal species, streptococcal species, and gram-negative aerobic bacteria are most commonly isolated [4–6]. Staphylococcal species are present 46% to 74% of the time, usually *Staphylococcus intermedius* [4,5,7,8].

Anaerobic bacteria also play a role in orthopedic infections. Isolation rates can be as high as 70%, but that might be site dependent, with the radius and/or ulna, mandible, and tympanic bulla commonly involved [1]. Anaerobic bacteria should be suspected in cases of grossly apparent infection with lack of growth on culture, infections secondary to disruption of tissues normally inhabited by anaerobic bacteria, or when inoculation from external sources has occurred [1,9–11]. Common isolates include *Bacteroides*, *Fusobacterium*, *Actinomyces*, *Clostridium* species, *Peptococcus* species, and *Peptostreptococcus* species [1,10,12].

Mycotic bone infections also occur but generally result from hematogenous spread [11]. Fungal organisms isolated from osseous infections include *Cryptococcus neoformans*, *Coccidioides immitis*, *Aspergillus* species, *Penicillium* species, *Blastomyces dermatitidis*, *Histoplasma capsulatum*, and *Phialemaenium* [13–18].

Staphylococci, streptococci, *Escherichia coli*, and *Pasteurella* species are commonly isolated from septic joints, with staphylococci being most prevalent [19,20]. *Borrelia burgdorferi*, bacterial L-forms, *Mycoplasma spumans*, *Mycobacterium*

E-mail address: lbubenik@vetmed.lsu.edu

0195-5616/05/$ – see front matter
doi:10.1016/j.cvsm.2005.05.001

tuberculosis, fungi, protozoa, and rickettsial organisms have also been implicated in infectious arthritis [21].

For diagnosis, infected tissue, direct sampling, or needle aspirates should be collected aseptically from the affected area for aerobic and anaerobic culture and for antimicrobial susceptibility testing. Aspiration alone resulted in an 86% isolation rate in one study [22]; however, other authors report less success [4,5]. Tissue culture or direct sampling is more likely to result in a positive culture. Culture of draining tracts should be avoided, because contaminants are usually isolated instead of the causative organism [23,24]. Blood cultures should be performed in animals with systemic disease [25]. In people with orthopedic infections and systemic disease, approximately 50% of blood cultures are positive with the causative organism [26]. In cases of aspergillosis, fungal hyphae can be seen microscopically in urine sediment and can be cultured from urine and synovium in some infected animals [13].

ANTIMICROBIAL THERAPY

Antibiotic penetration into bone and joint cavities and efficacy against the causative organism are necessary for resolution of infection. Penicillins and penicillin combination drugs, cephalosporins, and aminoglycosides readily penetrate normal and infected bone [27–31]. Staphylococci isolated from canine infections are often resistant to pure penicillins because of β-lactamase production, so β-lactamase–resistant drugs are more ideal [32]. Aminoglycosides lose some effectiveness in hypoxic and/or acidotic conditions and in the presence of white blood cells, so efficacy should be monitored during treatment [33]. Clindamycin penetrates normal bone and is useful for gram-positive and anaerobic osteomyelitis [34–36]. Fluoroquinolones also have good bone penetration and are beneficial for gram-negative infections [37]. Fluoroquinolones are not effective under anaerobic conditions and should be avoided in immature animals because of the potential deleterious effects on cartilage [38,39].

Synovial fluid and serum antibiotic kinetics are similar, with synovial fluid concentrations gradually increasing as serum concentrations rise, independent of the antibiotic administered [33,39]. The final synovial fluid concentration depends on the molecular size of the antibiotic and inflammation-dependent changes in synovial permeability [33,39]. Synovial fluid antibiotic concentrations decrease as joint inflammation resolves, but therapeutic antibiotic concentrations likely remain [40,41]. Antibiotic concentration within the joint is the same or higher with systemic administration when compared with intra-articular injection [42]. Furthermore, intra-articular injection of antibiotics can cause chemical synovitis with worsening of the pathologic process and should be avoided [43,44]. Tetracycline is recommended for those animals with infectious arthritis secondary to *Borrelia*, rickettsial infections, *Mycoplasma*, and bacterial L-forms [21,45].

Antibiotic choice is based on culture and antimicrobial susceptibility testing. Empiric therapy is used while culture and antimicrobial susceptibility is pending or when cultures fail to offer an appropriate therapeutic strategy. Care should be taken in antibiotic selection, however, because antimicrobial resistance of commonly isolated organisms is constantly changing. In one report, staphylococci showed 18% resistance to first-generation cephalosporins, although cephalosporins are commonly used antibiotics in the first line of defense against bone and joint infections [46].

Duration of antimicrobial therapy depends on the severity of the infection, but antibiotics should be continued for at least 2 weeks beyond radiographic and clinical resolution of infection, which typically requires weeks to months of therapy [33,47]. In cases of severe soft tissue destruction, free microvascular muscle flaps provide increased blood supply and delivery of antibiotics and healing factors to the wound bed [48]. Owners should be warned that treatment is likely to require long-term commitment and that it can be expensive.

Systemic antibiotic therapy is essential in the treatment of orthopedic infections. Although not effective at resolving orthopedic infections alone, local antibiotic therapy provides another means of treatment that may have some advantages when combined with systemic therapy [22,49–51]. Local antibiotic administration maintains a higher local drug concentration at the site of infection for a prolonged period [52,53] with reduced systemic toxicity [52–55]. Local delivery of antibiotics occurs mainly through temporary implantation of antibiotic-impregnated polymethylmethacrylate (AIPMMA) at the site of infection, but biodegradable delivery systems have also been investigated [56–59]. Local antibiotic delivery systems work by gradual release of antibiotics at the site of infection via antibiotic elution out of the implanted material. The antibiotic tissue concentration and elution rate depend on multiple factors, including the antibiotic used, cement configuration, type of antibiotic carrier, and tissue environment [49,53–55,60–63]. AIPMMA is often used in the form of preformed beads. The beads are placed at the site of infection and are left there for a duration based on the expected elution rate of the impregnated antibiotic. Beads can be serially replaced to maintain an adequate local antibiotic concentration, but implanted cement should ultimately be removed from the infected site because it can harbor bacteria and result in recurrent osteomyelitis [64].

IMAGING
Radiography is commonly used in the evaluation of osteomyelitis. Radiographs alone only have a sensitivity of 62.5% and a specificity of 57.1% for the diagnosis of osteomyelitis but are commonly used in conjunction with clinical signs to make a diagnosis [65]. For an acute infection, soft tissue swelling predominates without alteration in bone architecture [11]. With chronic infection, periosteal new bone proliferation, cortical bone resorption, cortical thinning, implant loosening, or bone sequestration might be apparent [2,4,5,11,24]. Osteolytic and productive changes can lag for 10 to 14 days after infection, so obtaining a second radiograph 1 to 2 weeks later might aid in the diagnosis of questionable cases [3]. Contrast radiography (fistulogram) can

be performed on draining tracts to help identify sequestra or foreign bodies [11]. Scintigraphy with technetium-99 methylene diphosphonate can provide early information regarding active bone or joint remodeling; however, it is not specific for infection [66,67]. MRI and CT can also aid in early diagnosis of osteomyelitis [68–70].

Radiographic changes associated with infectious arthritis include distention of the joint capsule, thickening of the synovial membrane, and widening of the joint space. With progression of disease, joint destruction, subchondral bone sclerosis, and fibrous or bony ankylosis can be seen [71]. Advanced imaging, such as CT, MRI, and scintigraphy, can also be useful in the diagnosis of joint infections [69,71].

ACUTE HEMATOGENOUS OSTEOMYELITIS

Clinical findings

Acute hematogenous osteomyelitis is not common and typically affects young animals, although animals at any age are at risk [4,5]. Osseous infection is seeded from infectious foci at a distant site in the body. Findings include soft tissue swelling over the affected site, moderate to severe lameness, inappetence, malaise, fever, or debilitation. The source of bone infection may or may not be found on examination.

Pathophysiology

Infection typically involves the metaphyseal region of the long bones, but diaphyseal infections can also occur [5,72]. Bacteria easily lodge in the metaphysis, where the endothelium of capillaries is discontinuous and blood flow slows as it reaches the metaphyseal veins [73,74]. After seeding the metaphysis, bacteria and activated platelets cause inflammation and thrombus formation, producing an ischemic environment that is conducive to bacterial proliferation [74]. Once infection is established, it is walled off by the immune response or it progresses [75]. With active infection, cellular debris, the in-flammatory cascade, and bacteria cause thrombosis, abscessation, and compromise of the blood supply. Sequestration of bone can occur when exudate reaches the outer cortex and elevates the periosteum, compromising cortical blood supply and devitalizing that portion of bone [74]. Draining tracts can also occur, although they more often develop in chronic infections [74]. Chronic osteomyelitis can result if the infection is walled off but not eliminated.

Diagnosis

A history of prior infection in conjunction with physical examination findings consistent with osteomyelitis is suggestive of septic seeding of the bone with bacteria. A complete blood cell count, biochemistry panel, and urinalysis might show other organ system involvement or be suggestive of infection. The results of such tests may not reveal anything of significance, however. Radiographs demonstrate only soft tissue swelling in the acute stage, but new bone production might become evident 2 to 3 weeks later [76]. Fine needle aspiration of fluctuant areas or surrounding tissues should be attempted to obtain an accurate diagnosis. The area should be aseptically prepared, and samples should be submitted for cytology, culture, and bacterial susceptibility testing. If systemic disease is present, blood cultures should also be performed. Gram staining of exudate might provide early information for treatment while awaiting culture results.

Treatment

Hematogenous osteomyelitis is best treated aggressively. A broad-spectrum bactericidal antimicrobial is administered intravenously for 3 to 5 days while awaiting culture and susceptibility results. Clinical response should be carefully monitored after treatment is initiated. A favorable initial response permits a change to oral antimicrobial administration within the first few days of therapy. Antimicrobial administration should be continued for at least 4 weeks and be based on culture and susceptibility results [77]. If the causative organism cannot be identified, continued antimicrobial administration is based on appropriate response to the initial therapeutic regimen. Fluid therapy, nutritional supplementation, and analgesics should be instituted as needed.

Some animals require surgery for complete resolution of disease. Palpable abscesses are drained, debrided, cultured, and lavaged. If debridement is adequate, closure over an active drain can be considered; however, if it is not adequate, the wound is left open and closed at a later time once the tissues appear healthy. Most animals respond favorably to treatment if antibiotic therapy is appropriate and the inciting cause is treated appropriately.

OSTEOMYELITIS FROM EXOGENOUS SOURCES

Exogenous bone infection occurs through direct inoculation (eg, bites, punctures, surgery), open fractures, foreign body migration, and gun shot wounds. Soft tissue injury, bone devitalization, surgical implants, instability of bone fragments, prolonged wound exposure, and immunosuppression increase the risk of bone infection, whereas normal bone is resistant [78,79].

Acute osteomyelitis

Clinical findings

Acute osteomyelitis is usually a complication of surgical fracture repair, and clinical signs are apparent 5 to 7 days after surgery. There is not a breed or sex predilection, but long bones are more often affected than axial bones, probably because of an increased predilection of fracture in long bones [2,4,5]. The surgical wound may be edematous, erythematous, and warm, and the limb is usually painful during manipulation. Animals are often febrile and have a substantial lameness. Although uncommon in the acute scenario, a draining tract might be present. Signs of systemic illness, such as inappetence and lethargy, might also be apparent [11].

Pathophysiology

The degree of soft tissue devitalization, fracture stability, type of fracture repair, organism virulence, and immune system competence influence the development of fracture site infection [2,11,78]. Trauma from fracture generation or surgery and implants applied during fracture repair disrupt blood supply and provide foreign material for bacterial adherence and proliferation [78]. Foreign bodies (including implants) decrease the quantity of bacteria needed to establish infection and provide a site for bacterial adherence that is sequestered from the immune system and antibiotics [78,80]. Moreover, the presence of dead bone at the fracture site substantially increases the risk of infection for virulent and nonvirulent strains of bacteria [81]. If bacteria gain access to the fracture site and these predisposing factors are present, the risk of infection is increased. Gun shots and bite wounds cause soft tissue injury and a means of bacterial inoculation. Furthermore, gun shots, migrating foreign bodies, and, occasionally, bites leave material behind that allow bacteria to evade host immune responses and proliferate [11].

Diagnosis

A history of recent fracture repair; an animal bite; evidence of foreign body migration; or a puncture wound and lameness, pain, heat, and swelling over the affected area suggest acute osteomyelitis of exogenous origin. Leukocytosis might be apparent on blood work, but evidence of systemic involvement is not common. Radiographs might demonstrate proliferative new bone and occasional gas in soft tissues, but soft tissue swelling might be the only radiographic sign. Bone sequestra can be present, but it can take several weeks for them to show up radiographically. Material obtained from fine needle aspiration of the involved site, directly from the affected sight via surgery, or from a draining tract is submitted for culture and susceptibility testing. Exudate from draining tracts often contains opportunistic organisms and not the offending organism, however [23,24].

Treatment

Aggressive early intervention is necessary for resolution and prevention of chronic osteomyelitis. If a fracture is present, it must be adequately stabilized. Loose implants must be removed. In some cases, external fixation can provide stability while minimizing soft tissue damage. Intravenous broad-spectrum bactericidal antibiotics are initially used. Antimicrobial protocols are modified pending culture, bacterial susceptibility results, and clinical response. Once a positive clinical response is noted, oral therapy can be continued at home. The duration of antibiotic administration varies, but it should be continued for at least 2 weeks beyond radiographic and clinical resolution of signs. For people with acute osteomyelitis, antibiotic administration for a minimum of 30 days is associated with a low rate of recurrence [82].

If foreign material is present, a fracture site is unstable, or abscessation and/or a draining tract is present, the affected site requires surgical exploration. The area is debrided and lavaged, and samples are obtained for culture and susceptibility testing. If possible, all foreign material is removed. If debridement is thorough and the tissues appear healthy, the wound is closed over an active drain with a low-pressure suction system. This drainage system is removed when fluid accumulation is minimal. Open wound management with delayed closure is necessary in some cases.

Many animals respond favorably to initial treatment if the inciting cause is eliminated and an appropriate antibiotic regimen is initiated and maintained [2,47]. Chronic osteomyelitis can develop if treatment is not effective.

Chronic osteomyelitis

Clinical findings

Animals suffering from chronic osteomyelitis usually present with an insidious lameness and varying degrees of pain at the fracture site. If an unstable fracture is present, the degree of fracture healing might influence the degree of lameness. Moderate to severe muscle atrophy is usually present in the affected limb. A draining tract is likely to be present. Owners might comment that drainage dissipates with antimicrobial administration only to return once antimicrobials are discontinued. Muscle fibrosis and contracture might also be apparent attributable to the effects of infection on the soft tissues [11]. Signs of systemic involvement are rare but can be present.

Pathophysiology

Chronic osteomyelitis develops from inadequate treatment of acute osteomyelitis or from hidden infections associated with implants, other foreign material, or bacterial isolation from the immune system through biofilm production [78,83,84]. Granulation and fibrous tissue can isolate devitalized bone (sequestra) and cause delayed healing or persistent infection [74,81]. Persistent infection is enhanced by the presence of metallic implants [78,80,85].

Diagnosis

A history of previous fracture repair, acute osteomyelitis, or chronic lameness, along with compatible physical examination findings, is sufficient to make a tentative diagnosis of chronic osteomyelitis. Radiographic signs include extensive bone remodeling with new bone production, lysis, and, often, the presence of a sequestrum [86]. Fine needle aspirates of affected tissues or samples obtained during surgery are submitted for culture and susceptibility testing. Fine needle aspiration might be less rewarding, because some bacteria adhere tightly to surrounding structures and do not exfoliate well [78,84,87]. If possible, antibiotics should be withheld for at least 24 hours before sample collection to improve yield [88].

Treatment

Chronic osteomyelitis is treated with surgery and appropriate antibiotic therapy [89]. Aggressive debridement of devitalized bone fragments and necrotic soft tissue, removal of sclerotic bone occluding the medullary canal, and removal of loose implants or foreign material are necessary to promote resolution [90]. The wound is closed primarily or over an active drain depending on tissue characteristics at the time of debridement. Multiple operations might be necessary to resolve infection in refractory cases [2].

Stabilization of an unstable fracture is essential. For amenable fractures, external fixators can be applied with minimal disruption of the blood supply and the added advantage of being easily removed [91]. If the soft tissues are healthy and the surgical procedure has consisted primarily of sequestrectomy and debridement of a fistulous tract, internal fixation can be considered [92,93]. Eventually, all implants require removal because they can harbor organisms and lead to recurrent osteomyelitis [80]. Bone grafting should be considered; however, delayed grafting might be necessary in excessively exudative wounds, because graft resorption can occur [7,75].

Nursing care is important in cases of chronic osteomyelitis because considerable muscle atrophy, fibrosis, or contracture can prevent return to function. Passive range-of-motion exercises on the affected limb are started immediately and continued several times daily until the animal is using its leg consistently. The animal should be encouraged to use the leg while ambulating. Pain medication is important to encourage weight bearing and limb use. Swimming and underwater treadmill activity can be beneficial.

A favorable response to treatment can occur in 90% of affected dogs, but recurrence is possible [2,47]. Complications of chronic osteomyelitis include refractory and/or recurrent osteomyelitis, nonunion, restricted joint motion, and loss of limb function. In severe cases with irreversible muscle damage and excessive joint stiffness, amputation might be necessary.

FUNGAL OSTEOMYELITIS
Clinical findings
Clinical presentation of animals suffering from fungal osteomyelitis is similar to that of animals suffering from bacterial osteomyelitis. Signs include lameness, soft tissue swelling, pain associated with the affected area, and the presence of draining tracts. Animals with fungal osteomyelitis often have disseminated disease with systemic signs such as general malaise, inappetence, respiratory compromise, lymphadenopathy, weight loss, and fever [13,94]. German Shepherd dogs may be overrepresented, possibly because of genetic factors involving altered immune function [13], but any age, breed, and sex can be affected.

Pathophysiology
Fungal organisms typically gain entrance to the body via inhalation, spread from the gastrointestinal tract, or direct inoculation with hematogenous dissemination thereafter [13,16–18,95–97]. Primary fungal osteomyelitis is rare [17].

Diagnosis
A diagnosis of fungal osteomyelitis is often made from cytologic or histologic evaluation of affected tissues. Cytology of affected areas mostly consists of pleocellular infiltration, including macrophages, lymphocytes, plasma cells, neutrophils, and multinucleated giant cells; lesions are pyogranulomatous in nature [94]. Fungal hyphae or intracellular organisms are often apparent on

preparations [13,16–18,95–97]. Special stains, such as Indian ink, periodic acid–Schiff, and silver nitrate stains, or treatment of preparations with 10% potassium hydroxide can improve visualization of organisms [94,95]. Serologic testing might be helpful to identify exposure [94]. Fungal culture is necessary for definitive diagnosis. Bone biopsy should be performed to obtain samples for culture and histopathologic examination.

Radiographic changes include soft tissue swelling, periosteal and endosteal bone proliferation, and bone lysis. Lesions are typically below the elbow and stifle but may be anywhere and must be differentiated from bone tumors [13,16–18,95–97].

A complete blood cell count and biochemistry profile are not specific for fungal disease, but findings include nonregenerative anemia, leukocytosis, hyperglobulinemia, and eosinophilia [13,16–18,95–97]. Fungal hyphae might be present in the urine of systemically ill patients [13].

Treatment

Treatment of fungal osteomyelitis is difficult and expensive. Animals require long-term antifungal therapy (months) and are treated at least a month beyond resolution of clinical signs [98]. Some animals require lifelong therapy [98] or amputation [95]. Antifungals include fluconazole, ketoconazole, amphotericin B, and itraconazole, but itraconazole is associated with fewer side effects [98]. The prognosis is guarded to poor for animals with systemic disease, although some animals respond to therapy. Recurrence is possible [18,98] and varies from 20% to 25% in cases of blastomycosis [98]. Histoplasmosis infection in cats often responds favorably to itraconazole [98].

SEPTIC ARTHRITIS

Septic arthritis results from hematogenous or exogenous joint contamination with bacteria. Exogenous infection results from penetrating injuries, surgical procedures, or intra-articular injections. Hematogenous infection occurs when bacteria from distant sites, such as the respiratory or digestive tract, umbilicus, urinary tract, or heart, localize in the joint [99]. Compromised synovial tissues secondary to preexisting disease [100] or conditions causing immunosuppression [21,100] predispose to joint infection.

Clinical findings

An infected joint is swollen and painful. The joint may be warm to the touch, and the animal is often severely lame or not weight bearing. Usually, only one joint is involved. Animals may or may not be febrile. Systemic signs are variable in cases of exogenous disease and not that common. In cases of hematogenous infection, however, systemic signs are likely to be present [45].

Feline calicivirus can produce acute arthritis in cats. In addition to fever, anorexia, depression, and oral ulcerations, cats affected with this syndrome exhibit acute swelling and pain of the distal joints and may be reluctant to move [101,102].

Pathophysiology

Bacterial infiltration into the joint results in synovial tissue edema, activation of the immune system, and initiation of the inflammatory cascade. Inflammation of the synovium, capillary rupture, and local areas of necrosis promote extravasation of fibrin, clotting factors, polymorphonuclear leukocytes, and proteinaceous serous fluid into the joint [103]. As a result, intra-articular pressure increases, potentially leading to ischemia, subluxation, or avascular necrosis. Activation of the inflammatory cascade results in release of lysosomal enzymes and enzyme byproducts that degrade cartilage, disrupt synovial fluid dynamics, and impair cartilage nutrition [103]. When combined with excessive joint motion, fragmentation of collagen fibrils and irreversible cartilage damage occur. Formation of granulation tissue within the joint contributes to joint destruction by penetrating and undermining the cartilage [104]. As the inflammatory process and infection progress and cartilage is destroyed, subchondral bone can also become involved [104]. Destruction of articular cartilage and degenerative joint changes combined with thickening and scaring of periarticular tissues lead to restricted joint motion and, in severe cases, loss of joint function. Early therapeutic intervention is imperative to decrease the severity of these joint changes [105,106].

Diagnosis

Definitive diagnosis of septic arthritis is based on aseptic arthrocentesis, followed by cytologic evaluation and culture and bacterial susceptibility testing of the synovial fluid. Abnormal findings include increased numbers of neutrophils (40,000 cells/mm^3 or greater), loss of fluid viscosity, presence of bacteria, and increased fluid turbidity. Direct culture of synovial fluid is not ideal because cultures are frequently negative [41,106]. To facilitate bacterial growth, synovial fluid is immediately placed into blood culture media at a 1:9 ratio. The synovial fluid–culture media samples are incubated for 24 hours at 37°C before being plated for identification of organisms [106]. Culture of synovial tissue has been reported to be more beneficial than culture of synovial fluid [19,45], but reports are conflicting in that experimental work has not shown the same [106]. Submission of synovial fluid on a culture swab should be carefully considered, because swabs have the potential to inhibit and absorb some organisms, resulting in a decreased yield [107], although success can be achieved using the technique [106]. Synovial fluid from cats with calicivirus infection can be normal or have elevated cell counts with a predominance of mononuclear cells; virus isolation is possible from synovial fluid and tissues of affected joints [102]. Polymerase chain reaction with DNA isolation can be useful in some cases of septic arthritis in which diagnosis is difficult, such as mycobacterial infections [108].

Early radiographic changes include joint effusion and soft tissue swelling. With progression of disease, bone lysis, joint surface irregularity, and subluxation can be seen. Nuclear scintigraphy provides earlier diagnostic information than conventional radiography, but positive joints do not specifically indicate infection [76,109,110].

Treatment

Therapy is directed at minimizing cartilage destruction. Antimicrobials are administered soon after samples for cytologic evaluation and culture have been obtained. Intravenous administration of a broad-spectrum bactericidal antimicrobial is indicated pending culture and bacterial susceptibility test results. Long-term antimicrobial administration is based on culture and bacterial susceptibility test results. If culture results are negative, antimicrobial therapy is continued based on a positive clinical response to treatment. Antimicrobials should be continued for a minimum of 4 weeks or at least 2 weeks beyond resolution of clinical signs.

Medical management consisting of appropriate antimicrobial therapy, passive range-of-motion exercises, and pain management can result in resolution of infection if the animal is treated aggressively and early in the course of disease [111]. Joint lavage is essential to remove cellular and enzymatic constituents in some cases, however. In young animals, decompression is particularly important to reduce pressure within the joint and preserve epiphyseal vascularity [103]. Needle aspiration and lavage do not adequately remove deleterious materials from the joint but can provide some benefit if surgical lavage is not an option [111]. Arthrotomy or arthroscopy with surgical debridement and copious lavage of the affected joint is indicated for postoperative joint infections, septic joints untreated for 72 hours or more, joints that have not responded to 72 hours of appropriate medical management, or joint infection secondary to penetrating wounds [39]. At the time of surgery, the joint is explored, debrided of necrotic debris, and lavaged with large volumes of isotonic solution. An entrance-exit joint flushing system allows for further lavage during the postoperative period and is considered for animals with severe infections and extensive tissue damage. Intra-articular drainage systems can be difficult to maintain, however, and open joint management is an effective alternative. Open joints and lavage systems should be managed sterilely, and the drains should be removed or the joint closed when drainage is minimal and less purulent. Joints with healthy appearing tissue after debridement and lavage are closed primarily at the time of surgery.

It is important to maintain joint mobility with passive range-of-motion activity yet to limit heavy weight-bearing exercise to prevent undue stress on the already weakened articular cartilage. Pain medication is imperative to facilitate joint mobility and animal comfort. Swimming or underwater treadmill activity would be beneficial.

The prognosis is variable and depends on the degree of cartilage destruction and duration of disease. Arthritis is expected after joint infection, but the severity and resulting disability are difficult to predict. Up to 50% of people suffer permanent joint dysfunction, and 75% have residual disabilities after treatment of septic arthritis [112,113]. Many animals recover with minimal deficits, but others suffer permanent joint dysfunction just as people do [20,111]. Furthermore, some animals have a residual lameness secondary to a continued immune response to lingering microbial antigens within the joint, although the infection has been eradicated [114]. These animals might respond to prednisolone therapy, but therapy should only be initiated after repeated negative joint cultures [21]. Calicivirus infection in kittens is usually self-limiting but can be associated with a 25% mortality rate in adult cats [101,102].

SUMMARY

Orthopedic infections can be expensive and challenging to treat. Parenteral antibiotic therapy is followed by long-term oral antibiotic administration. Surgical intervention is necessary in some cases for debridement of devitalized tissue and lavage. Fracture infections are difficult to manage and can require multiple operations to maintain fracture stability and tissue viability. Septic arthritis should be treated aggressively and early in the course of disease. Arthritis is expected after joint infection, but early treatment can minimize joint destruction. If appropriate treatment for orthopedic infections is instituted early, many animals have a functional outcome.

References

[1] Muir P, Johnson KA. Anaerobic bacteria isolated from osteomyelitis in dogs and cats. Vet Surg 1992;21(6):463–6.

[2] Braden TD. Posttraumatic osteomyelitis. Vet Clin North Am Small Anim Pract 1991; 21(4):781–811.

[3] Parker RB. Treatment of post-traumatic osteomyelitis. Vet Clin North Am Small Anim Pract 1987;17(4):841–56.

[4] Smith CW, Schiller AG, Smith AR, et al. Osteomyelitis in the dog: a retrospective study. J Am Anim Hosp Assoc 1978;14:589–92.

[5] Caywood DD, Wallace LJ, Braden TD. Osteomyelitis in the dog: a review of 67 cases. J Am Vet Med Assoc 1978;172(8):943–6.

[6] Griffiths GL, Bellenger CR. A retrospective study of osteomyelitis in dogs and cats. Aust Vet J 1979;55(12):587–91.

[7] Bardet JF, Hohn RB, Basinger R. Open drainage and delayed autogenous cancellous bone grafting for treatment of chronic osteomyelitis in dogs and cats. J Am Vet Med Assoc 1983;183(3):312–7.

[8] Hirsh DC, Smith TM. Osteomyelitis in the dog: microorganisms isolated and susceptibility to antimicrobial agents. J Small Anim Pract 1978;19:679–87.

[9] Dow SW, Jones RL, Adney WS. Anaerobic bacterial infections and response to treatment in dogs and cats: 36 cases (1983–1985). J Am Vet Med Assoc 1986;189(8):930–4.

[10] Johnson KA, Lomas GR, Wood AK. Osteomyelitis in dogs and cats caused by anaerobic bacteria. Aust Vet J 1984;61(2):57–61.

[11] Johnson KA. Osteomyelitis in dogs and cats. J Am Vet Med Assoc 1994;204(12):1882–7.

[12] Walker RD, Richardson DC, Bryant MJ, et al. Anaerobic bacteria associated with osteomyelitis in domestic animals. J Am Vet Med Assoc 1983;182(8):814–6.

[13] Day MJ, Penhale WJ, Eger CE, et al. Disseminated aspergillosis in dogs. Aust Vet J 1986;63(2):55–9.

[14] Legendre AM, Walker M, Buyukmihci N, et al. Canine blastomycosis: a review of 47 clinical cases. J Am Vet Med Assoc 1981;178(11):1163–8.

[15] Lomax LG, Cole JR, Padhye AA, et al. Osteolytic phaeohyphomycosis in a German shepherd dog caused by Phialemonium obovatum. J Clin Microbiol 1986;23(5):987–91.

[16] Shelton GD, Stockham SL, Carrig CB, et al. Disseminated histoplasmosis with bone lesions in a dog. J Am Anim Hosp Assoc 1982;18:143–6.

[17] Wigney DI, Allan GS, Hay LE, et al. Osteomyelitis associated with *Penicillium veruculosum* in a German shepherd dog. J Small Anim Pract 1990;31:449–52.

[18] Brearley MJ, Jeffery N. Cryptococcal osteomyelitis in a dog. J Small Anim Pract 1992; 33:601–4.

[19] Bennett D, Taylor D. Bacterial infective arthritis in the dog. J Small Anim Pract 1988;29: 207–30.

[20] Marchevsky AM, Read RA. Bacterial septic arthritis in 19 dogs. Aust Vet J 1999; 77(4):233–7.

[21] Bennett D, May C. Joint diseases of dogs and cats. In: Ettinger SJ, Feldman EC, editors. Textbook of veterinary internal medicine, vol. 2. Philadelphia: WB Saunders; 1995. p. 2032–77.

[22] Dernell W, Withrow S, Straw R, et al. Clinical response to antibiotic impregnated poly methyl methacrylate bead implantation of dogs with severe infections after limb sparing and allograft replacement—18 cases (1994–1996). Vet Comp Orthop Traumatol 1998;11:94–9.

[23] Mackowiak PA, Jones SR, Smith JW. Diagnostic value of sinus-tract cultures in chronic osteomyelitis. JAMA 1978;239(26):2772–5.

[24] Dernell WS. Treatment of severe orthopedic infections. Vet Clin North Am Small Anim Pract 1999;29(5):1261–74. [ix].

[25] Dunn JK, Dennis R, Houlton JEF. Successful treatment of two cases of metaphyseal osteomyelitis in the dog. J Small Anim Pract 1992;33:85–9.

[26] Waldvogel FA, Medoff G, Swartz MN. Osteomyelitis: a review of clinical features, therapeutic considerations and unusual aspects. N Engl J Med 1970;282(4): 198–206.

[27] Cunha BA, Gossling HR, Pasternak HS, et al. The penetration characteristics of cefazolin, cephalothin, and cephradine into bone in patients undergoing total hip replacement. J Bone Joint Surg Am 1977;59(7):856–9.

[28] Fitzgerald RH Jr. Antibiotic distribution in normal and osteomyelitic bone. Orthop Clin North Am 1984;15(3):537–46.

[29] Darouiche RO, Green G, Mansouri MD. Antimicrobial activity of antiseptic-coated orthopaedic devices. Int J Antimicrob Agents 1998;10(1):83–6.

[30] Hall BB, Fitzgerald RH Jr. The pharmacokinetics of penicillin in osteomyelitic canine bone. J Bone Joint Surg Am 1983;65(4):526–32.

[31] Rosin H, Rosin AM, Kramer J. Determination of antibiotic levels in human bone. I. Gentamicin levels in bone. Infection 1974;2(1):3–6.

[32] Love D. Antimicrobial susceptibility of Staphylococci isolated from dogs. Aust Vet Pract 1989;19(4):196–200.

[33] Hughes S, Fitzgerald RJ. Musculoskeletal infections. Chicago: Year Book Medical Publishers; 1987.

[34] Braden TD, Johnson CA, Gabel CL, et al. Physiologic evaluation of clindamycin, using a canine model of posttraumatic osteomyelitis. Am J Vet Res 1987;48(7):1101–5.

[35] Norden CW, Shinners E, Niederriter K. Clindamycin treatment of experimental chronic osteomyelitis due to Staphylococcus aureus. J Infect Dis 1986;153(5):956–9.

[36] Smilack JD, Flittie WH, Williams TW Jr. Bone concentrations of antimicrobial agents after parenteral administration. Antimicrob Agents Chemother 1976;9(1):169–71.

[37] Fong IW, Ledbetter WH, Vandenbroucke AC, et al. Ciprofloxacin concentrations in bone and muscle after oral dosing. Antimicrob Agents Chemother 1986;29(3):405–8.

[38] Paton JH, Reeves DS. Fluoroquinolone antibiotics. Microbiology, pharmacokinetics and clinical use. Drugs 1988;36(2):193–228.

[39] Wolfson JS, Hooper DC. Fluoroquinolone antimicrobial agents. Clin Microbiol Rev 1989;2(4):378–424.

[40] Bertone AL, Jones RL, McIlwraith CW. Serum and synovial fluid steady-state concentrations of trimethoprim and sulfadiazine in horses with experimentally induced infectious arthritis. Am J Vet Res 1988;49(10):1681–7.

[41] Bertone AL, McIlwraith CW, Jones RL, et al. Comparison of various treatments for experimentally induced equine infectious arthritis. Am J Vet Res 1987;48(3):519–29.

[42] Errecalde JO, Carmely D, Marino EL, et al. Pharmacokinetics of amoxicillin in normal horses and horses with experimental arthritis. J Vet Pharmacol Ther 2001;24(1):1–6.

[43] Goldenberg DL, Brandt KD, Cohen AS, et al. Treatment of septic arthritis: comparison of needle aspiration and surgery as initial modes of joint drainage. Arthritis Rheum 1975;18(1):83–90.

[44] Orsini JA. Strategies for treatment of bone and joint infections in large animals. J Am Vet Med Assoc 1984;185(10):1190–3.

[45] Budsberg S. Musculoskeletal infections. In: Greene C, editor. Infectious diseases of the dog and cat. 2nd edition. Philadelphia: WB Saunders; 1998. p. 555–67.

[46] Prescott JF, Hanna WJ, Reid-Smith R, et al. Antimicrobial drug use and resistance in dogs. Can Vet J 2002;43(2):107–16.

[47] Budsberg SD, Kemp DT. Antimicrobial distribution and therapeutics in bone. Compend Contin Educ Pract Vet 1990;12(12):1758–62.

[48] Basher A, Presnell KR. Muscle transposition as an aid in covering traumatic tissue over the canine tibia. J Am Anim Hosp Assoc 1987;23:617–28.

[49] Calhoun JH, Mader JT. Antibiotic beads in the management of surgical infections. Am J Surg 1989;157(4):443–9.

[50] Fitzgerald RH Jr. Experimental osteomyelitis: description of a canine model and the role of depot administration of antibiotics in the prevention and treatment of sepsis. J Bone Joint Surg Am 1983;65(3):371–80.

[51] Ostermann PA, Seligson D, Henry SL. Local antibiotic therapy for severe open fractures. A review of 1085 consecutive cases. J Bone Joint Surg Br 1995;77(1):93–7.

[52] Eckman JB Jr, Henry SL, Mangino PD, et al. Wound and serum levels of tobramycin with the prophylactic use of tobramycin-impregnated polymethylmethacrylate beads in compound fractures. Clin Orthop 1988;237:213–5.

[53] Klemm KW. Antibiotic bead chains. Clin Orthop 1993;295:63–76.

[54] Adams K, Couch L, Cierny G, et al. In vitro and in vivo evaluation of antibiotic diffusion from antibiotic-impregnated polymethylmethacrylate beads. Clin Orthop 1992;278:244–52.

[55] Wininger DA, Fass RJ. Antibiotic-impregnated cement and beads for orthopedic infections. Antimicrob Agents Chemother 1996;40(12):2675–9.

[56] Gerhart TN, Roux RD, Hanff PA, et al. Antibiotic-loaded biodegradable bone cement for prophylaxis and treatment of experimental osteomyelitis in rats. J Orthop Res 1993;11(2):250–5.

[57] Jacob E, Setterstrom JA, Bach DE, et al. Evaluation of biodegradable ampicillin anhydrate microcapsules for local treatment of experimental staphylococcal osteomyelitis. Clin Orthop 1991;267:237–44.

[58] Mackey D, Varlet A, Debeaumont D. Antibiotic loaded plaster of Paris pellets: an in vitro study of a possible method of local antibiotic therapy in bone infection. Clin Orthop 1982;167:263–8.

[59] Mehta S, Humphrey JS, Schenkman DI, et al. Gentamicin distribution from a collagen carrier. J Orthop Res 1996;14(5):749–54.

[60] Nijhof M, Dhert W, Tilman P, et al. Release of tobramycin from tobramycin-containing bone cement in bone and serum of rabbits. J Mater Sci 1997;8:799–802.

[61] Buchholz HW, Elson RA, Heinert K. Antibiotic-loaded acrylic cement: current concepts. Clin Orthop 1984;190:96–108.

[62] Fish DN, Hoffman HM, Danziger LH. Antibiotic-impregnated cement use in US hospitals. Am J Hosp Pharm 1992;49(10):2469–74.

[63] Popham GJ, Mangino P, Seligson D, et al. Antibiotic-impregnated beads. Part II: factors in antibiotic selection. Orthop Rev 1991;20(4):331–7.

[64] Tobias KM, Schneider RK, Besser TE. Use of antimicrobial-impregnated polymethyl methacrylate. J Am Vet Med Assoc 1996;208(6):841–5.

[65] Braden T, Tvedten H, Motosky U. The sensitivity and specificity of radiology and histopathology in the diagnosis of post-traumatic osteomyelitis. Vet Comp Orthop Traumatol 1989;3:98–103.

[66] Mandell GA. Imaging in the diagnosis of musculoskeletal infections in children. Curr Probl Pediatr 1996;26(7):218–37.

[67] Willis RB, Rozencwaig R. Pediatric osteomyelitis masquerading as skeletal neoplasia. Orthop Clin North Am 1996;27(3):625–34.

[68] Gold RH, Hawkins RA, Katz RD. Bacterial osteomyelitis: findings on plain radiography, CT, MR, and scintigraphy. AJR Am J Roentgenol 1991;157(2):365–70.

[69] Schlesinger AE, Hernandez RJ. Diseases of the musculoskeletal system in children: imaging with CT, sonography, and MR. AJR Am J Roentgenol 1992;158(4):729–41.

[70] Erdman WA, Tamburro F, Jayson HT, et al. Osteomyelitis: characteristics and pitfalls of diagnosis with MR imaging. Radiology 1991;180(2):533–9.

[71] Owens JM, Ackerman N. Roentgenology of arthritis. Vet Clin North Am Small Anim Pract 1978;8(3):453–64.

[72] Emmerson TD, Pead MJ. Pathological fracture of the femur secondary to haematogenous osteomyelitis in a weimaraner. J Small Anim Pract 1999;40(5):233–5.

[73] Whalen JL, Fitzgerald RH Jr, Morrissy RT. A histological study of acute hematogenous osteomyelitis following physeal injuries in rabbits. J Bone Joint Surg Am 1988; 70(9):1383–92.

[74] Kahn DS, Pritzker KP. The pathophysiology of bone infection. Clin Orthop 1973;96:12–9.

[75] Resnick C, Resnick D. Pyogenic osteomyelitis and septic arthritis. In: Traveras J, Ferucci J, editors. Radiology, diagnosis, imaging, intervention. Philadelphia: JB Lippincott; 1986. p. 1–15.

[76] Gupta NC, Prezio JA. Radionuclide imaging in osteomyelitis. Semin Nucl Med 1988;18(4):287–99.

[77] Waldvogel F. Acute osteomyelitis. In: Schlossberg D, editor. Orthopedic infection. New York: Springer-Verlag; 1988. p. 116–33.

[78] Gristina AG, Costerton JW. Bacterial adherence and the glycocalyx and their role in musculoskeletal infection. Orthop Clin North Am 1984;15(3):517–35.

[79] Scheman L, Janota M, Lewin P. The production of experimental osteomyelitis. JAMA 1941;117:1525–9.

[80] Smith MM, Vasseur PB, Saunders HM. Bacterial growth associated with metallic implants in dogs. J Am Vet Med Assoc 1989;195(6):765–7.

[81] Evans RP, Nelson CL, Harrison BH. The effect of wound environment on the incidence of acute osteomyelitis. Clin Orthop 1993;286:289–97.

[82] Fitzgerald RH Jr, Peterson LF, Washington JA, et al. Bacterial colonization of wounds and sepsis in total hip arthroplasty. J Bone Joint Surg Am 1973;55(6):1242–50.

[83] Marrie TJ, Costerton JW. Mode of growth of bacterial pathogens in chronic polymicrobial human osteomyelitis. J Clin Microbiol 1985;22(6):924–33.

[84] Mayberry-Carson KJ, Tober-Meyer B, Smith JK, et al. Bacterial adherence and glycocalyx formation in osteomyelitis experimentally induced with Staphylococcus aureus. Infect Immun 1984;43(3):825–33.

[85] Petty W, Spanier S, Shuster JJ, et al. The influence of skeletal implants on incidence of infection. Experiments in a canine model. J Bone Joint Surg Am 1985;67(8): 1236–44.

[86] Tumeh SS, Aliabadi P, Seltzer SE, et al. Chronic osteomyelitis: the relative roles of scintigrams, plain radiographs, and transmission computed tomography. Clin Nucl Med 1988;13(10):710–5.

[87] Geissler WB, Purvis JM. Hematogenous osteomyelitis and septic arthritis in children: a ten year review. J Miss State Med Assoc 1989;30(3):71–4.

[88] Hall BB, Rosenblatt JE, Fitzgerald RH Jr. Anaerobic septic arthritis and osteomyelitis. Orthop Clin North Am 1984;15(3):505–16.

[89] Nunamaker D. Osteomyelitis. In: Newton C, Nunamaker D, editors. Textbook of small animal orthopaedics. Philadelphia: JB Lippincott; 1985. p. 499–510.

[90] Nunamaker DM. Management of infected fractures. Osteomyelitis. Vet Clin North Am Small Anim Pract 1975;5(2):259–71.

[91] Egger E, Greenwood K. External skeletal fixation. In: Slatter D, editor. Textbook of small animal surgery. Philadelphia: WB Saunders; 1985. p. 1972–88.

[92] Kaltenecker G, Wruhs O, Quaicoe S. Lower infection rate after interlocking nailing in open fractures of femur and tibia. J Trauma 1990;30(4):474–9.

[93] Muir P, Johnson KA. Interlocking intramedullary nail stabilization of a femoral fracture in a dog with osteomyelitis. J Am Vet Med Assoc 1996;209(7):1262–4.

[94] Jang SS, Biberstein EL. Fungal diseases. In: Green C, editor. Infectious diseases of the dog and cat. 2nd edition. Philadelphia: WB Saunders; 1998. p. 349–57.

[95] Marcellin-Little DJ, Sellon RK, Kyles AE, et al. Chronic localized osteomyelitis caused by atypical infection with Blastomyces dermatitidis in a dog. J Am Vet Med Assoc 1996;209(11):1877–9.

[96] Moore AH, Hanna FY. Mycotic osteomyelitis in a dog following nasal aspergillosis. Vet Rec 1995;137(14):349–50.

[97] Wolf AM. Histoplasma capsulatum osteomyelitis in the cat. J Vet Intern Med 1987;1(4):158–62.

[98] Legendre AM. Antimicrobial therapy. In: Kirk R, editor. Current veterinary therapy, vol. XII. Philadelphia: WB Saunders; 1995. p. 327–31.

[99] Trotter GW, Mellwraith CW. Infectious arthritis in horses. Proceedings of the American Association of Equine Practitioners 1982;27:173–83.

[100] Gardner GC, Weisman MH. Pyarthrosis in patients with rheumatoid arthritis: a report of 13 cases and a review of the literature from the past 40 years. Am J Med 1990;88(5):503–11.

[101] Barr M, Olsen C, Scott F. Feline viral diseases. In: Ettinger SJ, Feldman EC, editors. Textbook of veterinary internal medicine, vol. 1. 4th edition. Philadelphia: WB Saunders; 1995. p. 409–39.

[102] Levy JK, Marsh A. Isolation of calicivirus from the joint of a kitten with arthritis. [see comments]. J Am Vet Med Assoc 1992;201(5):753–5.

[103] Asmar BI. Osteomyelitis in the neonate. Infect Dis Clin North Am 1992;6(1):117–32.

[104] Alderson M, Nade S. Natural history of acute septic arthritis in an avian model. J Orthop Res 1987;5(2):261–74.

[105] Blinkhorn RJ Jr, Strimbu V, Effron D, et al. 'Punch' actinomycosis causing osteomyelitis of the hand. Arch Intern Med 1988;148(12):2668–70.

[106] Montgomery RD, Long IR Jr, Milton JL, et al. Comparison of aerobic culturette, synovial membrane biopsy, and blood culture medium in detection of canine bacterial arthritis. Vet Surg 1989;18(4):300–3.

[107] Carr A. Infectious arthritis in dogs and cats. Veterinary Medicine 1997;786–97.

[108] Canvin JM, Goutcher SC, Hagig M, et al. Persistence of Staphylococcus aureus as detected by polymerase chain reaction in the synovial fluid of a patient with septic arthritis. Br J Rheumatol 1997;36(2):203–6.

[109] Demopulous G, Bleck EE, McDougull IR. Role of radionuclide imaging in the diagnosis of acute osteomyelitis. J Pediatr Orthop 1988;8:558.

[110] Hoffer P, Newmann R. Diagnostic nuclear medicine. Baltimore: Williams & Wilkins; 1988.

[111] Fitch RB, Hogan TC, Kudnig ST. Hematogenous septic arthritis in the dog: results of five patients treated nonsurgically with antibiotics. J Am Anim Hosp Assoc 2003;39(6):563–6.

[112] Cooper C, Cawley MI. Bacterial arthritis in an English health district: a 10 year review. Ann Rheum Dis 1986;45(6):458–63.
[113] Meijers KA, Dijkmans BA, Hermans J, et al. Non-gonococcal infectious arthritis: a retrospective study. J Infect 1987;14(1):13–20.
[114] Dow SW, Lappin MR. Immunopathologic consequences of infectious disease. In: Breitschwerdt E, editor. Kirk's current veterinary therapy XII—small animal practice. Philadelphia: WB Saunders; 1995. p. 554–60.

Vet Clin Small Anim 35 (2005) 1111–1135

VETERINARY CLINICS
SMALL ANIMAL PRACTICE

ELSEVIER
SAUNDERS

Developmental Orthopedic Disease

Jennifer Demko, DVM, Ron McLaughlin, DVM, DVSc*

Department of Clinical Sciences, College of Veterinary Medicine, Mississippi State University,
Mississippi State, MS 39762, USA

D
evelopmental orthopedic diseases (DODs) are a common cause of
lameness and pain in young dogs. A thorough knowledge of the
patient's signalment and history and a complete physical examination
are necessary to localize the disease, establish a list of differential diagnoses, and
develop a diagnostic plan. A thorough understanding of the disease etiology,
pathophysiology, and progression is needed to recommend the appropriate
medical and surgical treatments.

HYPERTROPHIC OSTEODYSTROPHY

Signalment

Hypertrophic osteodystrophy (HOD) is an idiopathic disease that affects
rapidly growing large- and giant-breed dogs between 2 and 8 months of age [1–
4]. Although there is no known sex predilection, male dogs are overrepresented
in some reports [4–8]. Breeds found to have a higher incidence of HOD include
German Shepherds, Irish Setters, Weimeraners, Great Danes, and Chesapeake
Bay Retrievers [1–4].

Etiology and pathogenesis

The etiology of HOD is unknown. Reported potential causes include infection
(canine distemper virus and *Escherichia coli*), hypovitaminosis C, oversupple-
mentation with vitamins and minerals, vascular abnormalities, and genetics [4–
8]. Lesions similar to those of HOD have been experimentally produced in
dogs fed a free-choice diet high in protein, calcium, and calories [9].

Histologically, there is initially necrosis of the capillary loops that invade the
cartilage model of the metaphyseal physis. Congestion and edema occur in the
extraperiosteal soft tissues surrounding the metaphysis, followed by formation of a cuff of metaplastic cartilage and bone in the region [10]. Other
histopathologic changes that may occur in dogs with HOD that die after
a period of sustained high fever and systemic signs include interstitial
pneumonia and mineralization of soft tissues (lung, spleen, kidney, aorta, and

*Corresponding author. E-mail address: mclaughlin@cvm.msstate.edu (R. McLaughlin).

0195-5616/05/$ – see front matter
doi:10.1016/j.cvsm.2005.05.002

endocardium) [10]. In some dogs, viral inclusions resembling those of canine distemper virus have been observed in macrophages in the suppurative physeal lesions [10].

Clinical signs

Clinical signs of HOD include the acute onset of lethargy, reluctance to walk, mild to severe lameness, and generalized pain. The metaphyseal areas of affected long bones are swollen, firm, painful, and warm to the touch. These signs are most commonly observed in the distal radius, ulna, and tibia, although the ribs, mandible, scapula, and metacarpal bones may also be affected [3,6,11,12]. The lesions are usually bilateral and symmetric [13]. Systemic signs can include severe anorexia, weight loss, fever, and depression [9]. Death occurs in rare cases, usually caused by prolonged hyperthermia, euthanasia attributable to pain, long-term recumbency, anorexia, or general morbidity associated with the disease [14,15].

Diagnosis

The diagnosis of HOD is based on physical examination and radiographic findings. Lesions are most commonly seen in the distal radius, ulna, and tibia and have been reported in the femur. Dogs affected with HOD typically present with lameness, fever, and pain in the metaphyseal region of the long bones. Depression and anorexia are common. Radiographically, a radiolucent region (Fig. 1) is observed in the metaphysis parallel to the physis and is often referred to as a "double physeal line" [1–4]. Metaphyseal sclerosis, irregular widening of the physis, subperiosteal and extraperiosteal new bone formation may also be evident radiographically [9].

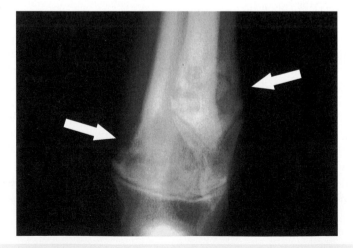

Fig. 1. Craniocaudal radiographic view of the distal radius and ulna of a dog with HOD. Arrows identify radiolucent regions in the metaphyses parallel to the growth plates ("double physeal line").

Treatment

Treatment of HOD consists of supportive care to maintain hydration, prevent decubital ulcers, and control pain. Nonsteroidal anti-inflammatory drugs (NSAIDs) are used to control pain in most cases, although corticosteroids have been used in unresponsive patients. A decrease in caloric intake may also be helpful in fast-growing dogs. Vitamin C and D supplementation has been described, but most reports indicate that such supplementation is not beneficial and may increase the risk of dystrophic calcification. Severe cases of HOD may require blood cultures to rule out septicemia. Broad-spectrum antibiotics are indicated with positive culture results [16].

Prognosis

HOD is usually a self-limiting disease with a good prognosis in uncomplicated cases. Permanent bony changes or growth plate abnormalities may occur in some cases, however. In severe cases, the prognosis is guarded, because systemic metabolic disease or secondary bacteremia causing tissue infections can lead to death or euthanasia. Specific vaccination protocols have been recommended (particularly for use in Weimaraners) using separate vaccines for canine distemper virus, parvovirus, and adenovirus or using killed vaccines in place of modified-live vaccines [17,18]. These protocols are thought to avoid the possible cause of vaccine-induced HOD.

PANOSTEITIS

Signalment

Panosteitis is an acquired self-limiting inflammatory condition of undetermined cause that affects the diaphyseal and metaphyseal regions of the long bones of large-breed dogs from 5 to 18 months of age. It is rarely seen in older animals. German Shepherds, Doberman Pinschers, Golden Retrievers, Saint Bernards, Labrador Retrievers, and Basset Hounds are among the overrepresented breeds affected with panosteitis, although it may occur in other breeds [9]. The disease affects male dogs more frequently than female dogs [9,19,20].

Etiology and pathogenesis

The etiology of panosteitis is unknown. Histologically, there is increased osteoblastic and fibroblastic activity affecting the endosteum, periosteum, and marrow of affected sites, resulting in fibrosis and connective tissue replacement of the normal medullary cavity. Leakage of protein-rich fluid from congested medullary vessels and secondary formation of haphazard trabecular systems occur. Pain is likely caused by medullary hypertension and congestion or stimulation of pain receptors in the periosteum. There is no evidence of inflammatory cell exudates, necrosis, or neoplasia [21].

Clinical signs

Clinical signs of panosteitis include acute lameness, with or without a history of trauma. Dogs are typically presented for an acute shifting leg lameness, lethargy, and pain that is cyclic and recurrent. Anorexia and fever may also be present. Pain is palpated along the diaphysis of long bones, especially the humerus, femur, and proximal radius and ulna [19,22]. Signs often resolve after several days or in 1 to 2 weeks; however, recurrence is common up to 18 months of age [9].

Diagnosis

The diagnosis of panosteitis is based on physical examination and radiographic findings. Early radiographic evidence of panosteitis includes an increased opacity of the medullary canal of long bones, usually near the nutrient foramen [13,23]. Blurring of the trabecular pattern and increased opacity of the endosteal surface of the medullary cavity are observed [19]. As the disease progresses, the medullary opacities become more delineated and begin to coalesce (Fig. 2). In 15% to 25% of cases, a smooth periosteal reaction occurs, giving the cortex a thicker appearance. Interestingly, radiographic signs may not always correlate with clinical lameness and may not be observed in early or mild cases of panosteitis. Radiographic lesions may occur in multiple bones simultaneously. Nuclear scintigraphy may aid in the diagnosis of cases of panosteitis in which radiographic signs are absent.

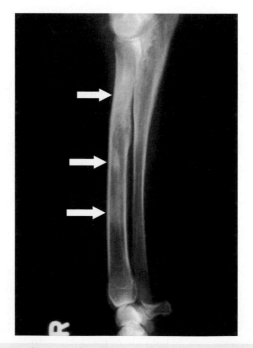

Fig. 2. Lateral radiographic view of the radius and ulna of a dog with panosteitis. Arrows identify areas of increased medullary opacity within the radius.

Treatment
Panosteitis is a self-limiting disease, and therapy consists of exercise restriction, weight reduction, and NSAIDs for pain management [13].

Prognosis
The prognosis for patients with panosteitis is excellent, and signs typically resolve by 18 to 20 months of age [24,25]. Secondary complications are rare [21,22]. In some dogs, intermittent lameness may occur for 6 to 18 months or longer and may shift to other limbs [21,22].

OSTEOCHONDROSIS
Signalment
Osteochondrosis (OC) is commonly observed in rapidly growing, large- and giant-breed, male dogs, typically between 5 and 10 months of age [26–31]. Puppies from predisposed breeds are typically large, have rapid growth rates, and are often on high planes of nutrition. The disease is most common in dogs that reach an adult weight of greater than 20 kg and tends to occur during periods of rapid growth. Puppies from small breeds of dogs are rarely affected with OC [27,32]. Male dogs are more commonly affected than female dogs [27,30,31]. The incidence of bilateral disease is reported to range from 20% to 85%, depending on the joint involved [26–33]. Right and left limbs are equally affected.

Etiology and pathogenesis
OC is a disturbance in the process of endochondral ossification in a focal area of a developing articular surface centered at the osteochondral junction. The cartilage in the affected site fails to undergo physiologic calcification and replacement by bone, leaving a thickened focal area of degenerative cartilage. This area of necrotic cartilage and fibrous tissue is vulnerable to shearing forces encountered during normal weight bearing and may become dislodged from the underlying bone, forming a flap (Fig. 3). This lesion is referred to as osteochondritis dissecans (OCD). When a flap forms, cartilage degradation products reach the synovial fluid, causing synovitis, effusion, joint pain, and lameness. The resultant flap of cartilage may remain within the defect or may become dislodged. Cartilage flaps that remain in the defect may reattach to the underlying subchondral bone, or the flap may break free, forming joint mice. Joint mice may be resorbed in synovial recesses or remain in the joint, causing synovitis and osteoarthritis (OA). The cause of OC has not been determined, but a multifactoral complex of factors, including genetics, rapid growth, overnutrition and excess dietary calcium, trauma, ischemia, and hormonal influences, has been implicated [34–36].

The shoulder (caudal humeral head) is the most frequently involved joint in dogs; however, the disease is also seen in the elbow (medial portion of the humeral condyle), stifle (lateral condyle of the femur), and hock (plantar aspect of the medial trochlear ridge). OC has also been reported in the medial femoral condyle, dorsal aspect of the lateral trochlear ridge and head of the femur,

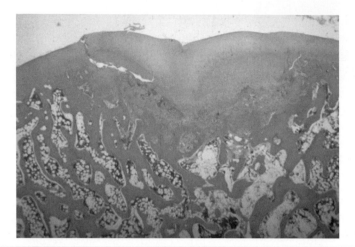

Fig. 3. Microscopic view of an OC lesion in the dog. Note the area of thickened articular cartilage separating the lesion from the underlying subchondral bone.

dorsal rim of the acetabulum, scapular glenoid cavity, and cervical vertebrae [35,37,38].

Clinical signs

The most common clinical sign is mild to moderate unilateral lameness, even with bilateral disease. The lameness is usually gradual in onset, and it improves with rest and worsens with exercise. Pain is elicited on palpation of affected joints. Stiffness and reduced range of motion may be present. Joint effusion may be palpable in some joints affected with OC. Muscle atrophy may be present, particularly in more chronic cases.

Diagnosis

A presumptive diagnosis of OC is based on the history and physical examination findings, but radiographs are necessary to confirm the diagnosis and should be taken bilaterally. OC typically appears radiographically as subchondral bone radiolucency or flattening [30,39,40]. Joint effusion or an increase in joint space may also be observed. If mineralized, cartilage flaps or joint mice may be visible radiographically. The most useful radiographic views for the diagnosis of OC depend on the joint involved. Other diagnostic techniques useful in the diagnosis of OC include arthroscopy, CT, and contrast arthrography.

Scapulohumeral joint

OC lesions are most commonly located on the caudal central aspect of the humeral head and visualized on mediolateral radiographs [30,39,40].

Cubital joint
OC lesions are typically located on the medial aspect of the humeral condyle and visualized on mediolateral, flexed mediolateral, and craniocaudal (elbow flexed 90° plus slight medial rotation) radiographic views [41–44].

Stifle joint
OC lesions usually appear on craniocaudal and lateral radiographic projections as a flattening of the subchondral bone of the lateral (96%) or medial (4%) femoral condyle. The medial aspect of the lateral femoral condyle is the most common location reported [45–47].

Tibiotarsal joint
Most (79%) tarsal OCD lesions involve the medial trochlear ridge of the talus [48]. Eighty percent of medial ridge lesions occur on the plantar aspect of the ridge. Twenty-one percent of tarsal OCD lesions involve the lateral trochlear ridge (70% of these lesions are on the dorsal aspect of the ridge) [40,49,50]. Approximately 90% of the dogs with lateral trochlear ridge lesions are Rottweilers [51]. Radiographic evaluation should include standard lateral, flexed lateral, and dorsoplantar views of both tarsi. Additional views are also helpful, including a craniocaudal view of the proximal trochlear ridges, a dorsolateral-plantomedial oblique view (D45°L-PLMO), and a dorsomedial-plantolateral oblique view (D45°M-PLLO) [52–54].

Treatment
Conservative therapy and surgery have been advocated for treatment of OC in dogs. Recommended treatment varies according to the joint affected, severity and chronicity of the lesion, clinician's experience, and financial restraints of the client.

Shoulder
Conservative treatment of shoulder OC may be warranted for dogs less than 7 months of age with mild lesions radiographically and no clinical pain or joint mice. Conservative therapy consists of strict rest for up to 6 weeks, restricted diet, NSAIDS, OA disease–modifying agents, and analgesics. Alterations in the diet include decreasing caloric intake, and stopping calcium supplementation may also be indicated [55]. If lameness persists for more than 4 to 6 weeks, surgery should be performed [56].

Surgery is recommended in dogs if a flap is present, the dog has been lame for more than 6 weeks, the dog is older than 8 months of age, a joint mouse is evident on radiographs, or the lesion is large. Surgical treatment provides a more rapid return to function and minimizes the development of OA. Arthroscopy is the preferred surgical treatment because it is less invasive and allows a more rapid return to limb function [29,57,58]. Whether an arthrotomy or arthroscopy is performed, the goal of surgery is to remove the cartilage flap or joint mice, remove cartilage in the periphery of the lesion that is not adhering to the underlying tissue, and stimulate defect healing. Healing of the defect requires bleeding from the subchondral bone to bring in mesenchymal cells and a fibrin clot [59]. Fibrocartilage eventually fills the defect. This bleeding can be induced by curettage, forage, or abrasion arthroplasty.

Elbow

Treatment of elbow OCD may include medical management or surgery. Surgical therapy involves removal of the cartilaginous flap with or without curettage of the defect bed. Several surgical techniques exist, but most surgeons prefer a medial approach and arthrotomy. Arthroscopic techniques are becoming more popular and allow exploration of the entire joint, removal of the cartilage flap, and forage or curettage of the defect [59,60]. Whenever possible, arthroscopic treatment is preferred.

Stifle

Medical management of stifle OCD is most successful in patients with mild lameness and only a small subchondral lesion evident radiographically. Surgical treatment is preferred in patients with persistent lameness, joint mice, or larger radiographic lesions. Arthrotomy or arthroscopy may be used to explore the joint, excise the cartilage flap and joint mice, and promote healing of the defect [61–64].

Hock

Medical management for tarsal OCD is recommended in older dogs with severe degenerative changes. Although most reports suggest that surgical intervention is preferred for treating tarsal OC, two recent studies found no significant differences in long-term outcome between joints treated medically and those treated surgically [64,65]. This is likely to be particularly true in dogs with chronic disease and significant OA. Surgical exploration and removal of the cartilage flap or osteochondral fragment can allow ingrowth of fibrocartilage from the underlying subchondral bone. Early intervention with a minimally invasive approach is preferred. Once the lesion is exposed, the cartilage flap or osteochondral fragment is excised. Overall function is better with minimal curettage. Arthroscopy of the tarsus has also been described for evaluation and diagnosis of tarsal diseases [66–68]. Arthroscopic removal of OCD fragments is possible in the dorsal aspect but can be difficult on the plantar aspect of the talus [67].

Prognosis

The prognosis after treatment of OC depends on the affected joint and whether medical or surgical treatment is used.

Shoulder

The prognosis after surgical treatment of shoulder OCD is good to excellent. Mild OA often develops in the operated shoulder over time, although lameness typically resolves and limb function is good [27]. Older dogs with chronic lameness and OA have a more guarded prognosis; however, most dogs return to normal function within 4 to 8 weeks after surgery.

Elbow

The prognosis for medical or surgical treatment of elbow OCD is guarded. Progression of secondary degenerative joint disease is common after medical management. Early surgical treatment of the OCD lesion does decrease lameness but may not prevent the progression of OA.

Stifle

The prognosis for dogs with stifle OC is guarded to fair. Progression of OA is common even after surgery. The severity of OA present before surgery, the size and location of the defect, and the quality of postoperative physical therapy all affect the long-term prognosis.

Hock

The prognosis for OC of the tarsus after conservative therapy is guarded. Most dogs have intermittent lameness and moderate progression of OA. After surgery, OA is likely and often requires medical therapy to control pain and lameness. Despite the progression of OA noted radiographically after surgery, many dogs are clinically improved. Nevertheless, the prognosis remains guarded, because joint pain and lameness may recur as the OA progresses. Recovery is faster in dogs with lesions involving the non–weight-bearing dorsal aspect of the lateral trochlear ridge [69]. Several factors may influence the success of medical and surgical treatment, including the age of the dog, presence of OA, size of the osteochondral defect, presence of joint instability, site of the lesion, and whether the lesions are unilateral or bilateral.

LEGG-CALVÉ-PERTHES DISEASE
Signalment
Legg-Calvé-Perthes Disease (LCPD), or avascular necrosis of the femoral head, is a developmental condition that occurs in primarily toy- and miniature-breed dogs [70–72]. Most patients are 4 to 11 months of age, and male and female dogs are equally represented. LCPD is reportedly bilateral in 12% to 16% of cases [70–73].

Etiology and pathogenesis
The etiology of femoral head necrosis in patients with LCPD is unknown. Numerous suspected causes have been investigated, including infection, trauma, metabolic and hormonal imbalances, vascular abnormalities, and genetics. The normal femoral head receives its blood supply from epiphyseal vessels that enter the epiphysis near the joint capsule insertion. Compromise of these vessels may cause ischemic insult to the epiphyseal spongiosa and its marrow elements. Synovitis or a sustained abnormal limb position may cause sufficient increases in intra-articular pressure to collapse fragile veins and deprive the femoral head of blood flow, resulting in regional or generalized necrosis [70,71]. Initially, the necrotic bone remains mechanically sound and continues to support the articular cartilage. Over time, however, the subchondral bony plate and overlying cartilage collapse, leading to a loss of

normal contour of the femoral head and secondary OA [70–73]. In cases of LCPD, transient or temporary vascular compromise rather than a permanent vascular insult is suspected, because reparative fibrosis and osteoblastic activity can be seen histologically after the initial ischemic phase of the disease [74]. In human beings, LCPD is thought to be inherited [74]. LCPD is also an inherited condition in Manchester Terriers [75].

Clinical signs

Clinical signs of LCPD are typically seen between 4 and 11 months of age. Most dogs have an acute onset of non–weight-bearing lameness or an intermittent subtle lameness [70–73]. Recent trauma may be reported by the owners. Other signs of LCPD include hip pain, crepitus of the hip during palpation, and muscle atrophy.

Diagnosis

The diagnosis of LCPD is based on history, physical examination, and radiographic findings. Early radiographic changes include increased radiopacity of the lateral epiphyseal area of the femoral head and focal bony lysis as resorption of the bony trabeculae progresses [74]. Later, flattening and a mottled appearance of the femoral head, collapse and thickening of the femoral neck, and potential femoral neck fractures can be seen on radiographs (Fig. 4) [9]. Degenerative joint disease and atrophy of the thigh muscles also become increasingly apparent later in the disease.

Treatment

Conservative and surgical treatment options have been reported for LCPD. Conservative therapy consists of rest, limited exercise, appropriate nutrition, and NSAIDs for analgesia. Published reports indicate that lameness resolves in less than 25% of affected dogs managed conservatively [72,73,76]. The preferred treatment for LCPD is femoral head and neck excisional arthroplasty. Surgery alleviates pain and lameness in 84% to 100% of patients regardless of age and progression of the disease [77].

Prognosis

The prognosis for a return to normal function is good to excellent in dogs that have surgery to remove the femoral head and neck. After surgery, passive range-of-motion exercises and controlled active exercise are encouraged to promote the creation of functional pseudoarthrosis. The degree of muscle atrophy present in the limb before surgery can affect the prognosis for limb function. Continue lameness is expected for patients that do not have surgery or if surgery is inadequate. Fracture of the femoral neck may occur in untreated patients. Proper technique in removing the femoral head and neck is critical for long-term success.

HIP DYSPLASIA

Signalment

Canine hip dysplasia (HD) most commonly affects large-breed dogs but is also seen in many small-breed dogs and cats [78–80]. Most dogs show clinical signs

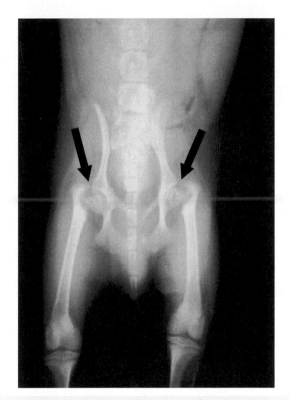

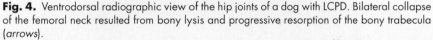

Fig. 4. Ventrodorsal radiographic view of the hip joints of a dog with LCPD. Bilateral collapse of the femoral neck resulted from bony lysis and progressive resorption of the bony trabecula (*arrows*).

of hip pain and lameness between 4 and 10 months of age. Many dogs are presented for treatment of HD after reaching skeletal maturity because of OA, however. Retrievers, Rottweilers, German Shepherds, and Saint Bernards are among the commonly affected breeds [78–80].

Etiology and pathogenesis

HD is a common skeletal developmental defect produced by a genetic predisposition to subluxation of the immature hip joint. Joint laxity is the initiating cause of dysplasia and leads to subluxation and poor congruence between the femoral head and the acetabulum. Abnormal forces develop across the joint that interfere with normal development and overload areas of articular cartilage. Over time, degeneration of the joint occurs. Numerous factors influence the development and progression of HD, including genetics, rapid weight gain in growing animals, a high nutrition level, and pelvic muscle mass.

Clinical signs

HD usually affects both hips, although one hip may appear more severely affected than the other. In many cases, dogs are presented for lameness in only one hind limb. Clinical signs of HD vary and may include decreased activity, difficulty in rising, reluctance to run or climb stairs, intermittent hind limb lameness, "bunny hopping," swaying gait, narrow stance, hip pain, atrophy of the thigh muscles, hypertrophy of the shoulder muscles, crepitus, and reduced hip joint motion. Joint laxity (detected clinically by a positive Ortolani sign) is characteristic of early HD; however, joint laxity may no longer be present in chronic cases because of periarticular fibrosis. In many cases, early signs are overlooked by owners and the dogs may not be presented for veterinary care until late in the disease when OA is severe.

Diagnosis

The diagnosis of HD is based on physical examination and radiographic findings. Physical examination typically reveals hip pain and a reduced range of motion. Most dogs are in pain on extension and abduction of the hip joint. Gait abnormalities are often observed and usually worsen with exercise.

Radiographic findings consistent with HD include hip joint laxity (subluxation) or secondary morphometric and degenerative changes within the joint [81]. Early in the disease, the shape of the acetabulum and femoral head is normal and the primary radiographic finding is joint incongruity. Identification of this joint laxity is essential to the early diagnosis of HD. Joint subluxation may be observed subjectively on a ventrodorsal hip-extended radiographic view of the pelvis [82,83]. The degree of subluxation can be quantified by measuring the Norberg angle (angle formed by a line drawn from the center of the femoral head to the cranial acetabular rim and a line drawn between the centers of the two femoral heads) or by calculating the percentage coverage of the femoral head by the acetabulum. Unfortunately, the magnitude of joint subluxation observed on ventrodorsal hip-extended radiographs is positionally dependent and can vary significantly in sequential radiographs obtained in the same dog. Additionally, the twisting of the joint capsule that occurs when the dog is placed in this position can mask the presence of joint laxity [84].

Distraction radiography provides a more sensitive means of identifying and measuring hip joint laxity. With the PennHip radiographic technique, the dog is positioned in dorsal recumbency with the femurs in a neutral position [85,86]. Distraction is created by placing a wedge between the dog's thighs and applying a medially directed force to the stifles. The distance the femoral head moves out of the acetabulum is measured to obtain a "distraction index," which is a measure of the passive laxity present in the joint. Measurement of the distraction index has been shown to be a reliable predictor of the eventual development of OA in lax hip joints. Another distraction radiographic technique is the dorsolateral subluxation (DLS) test. The dog is positioned in sternal recumbency with the knees flexed and adducted so that the femurs are perpendicular to the table surface [87,88]. With the hind limbs in this kneeling position, weight bearing is simulated and the femoral head subluxates dorsolaterally when laxity is present.

In more chronic cases of HD, radiographic changes indicative of joint degeneration and remodeling can be seen [81]. As abnormal forces continue to act on the lax hip joint, the acetabulum becomes shallow and the femoral head begins to flatten. Osteophytes form at the joint margins and are apparent radiographically as new bone production. The acetabular margin becomes irregular, and the femoral neck becomes thicker as the osteophytes are formed. Sclerosis of the subchondral bone develops and is often most apparent on the craniodorsal acetabular rim. Fibrosis and increased density of the periarticular soft tissues are also apparent radiographically. Because of periarticular fibrosis, joint laxity may no longer be a major component of the disease in chronic HD.

Treatment

Medical and surgical treatments have been used for HD in young dogs (Table 1). Medical treatment typically includes weight control or weight loss, physical therapy and exercise control, NSAIDs, and OA disease–modifying agents [89–99]. Medical therapy is quite successful in many cases.

Table 1
Considerations when selecting treatment for hip dysplasia

Treatment	Patient age	Patient size	Criteria	Complications
Medical therapy	Any age	Any size	Clinical signs Response to therapy	Progressive OA Gastrointestinal/renal complications
JPS	3–4 months	Any size	Age No OA Hip laxity	Narrowing of pelvic canal
TPO	Less than 10 months	Limited by availability of plate sizes	No OA Hip laxity Clinical signs present	Implant failure Infection Narrowing of pelvic canal
THA	After skeletal maturity (older than 10–12 months)	Limited by availability of implant size	Clinical signs Unresponsive to medical therapy No signs of infection (teeth, ears, skin)	Implant failure/luxation Infection Aseptic loosening Femoral fracture
FHNE	Any age	Any size (best <20 kg)	Clinical signs Unresponsive to medical therapy THA not possible or salvage	Gait abnormality Infection

Abbreviations: FHNE, femoral head and neck excision; JPS, juvenile pubic symphysiodesis; OA, osteoarthritis; THA, total hip arthroplasty; TPO, triple pelvic osteotomy.

Surgical techniques used to treat HD depend on the size and age of the dog, the amount of OA present, cost, and clinician preference. In young dogs with hip joint laxity and no OA, a triple pelvic osteotomy (TPO) is often recommended [100–103]. A TPO is a corrective surgical procedure that reorients the acetabulum to establish congruity between the femoral head and acetabulum. It increases acetabular coverage of the femoral head to eliminate subluxation and improve joint stability. To be successful, the procedure must be performed early in the disease process, before OA changes develop and while the remodeling capability exists to allow development of a more congruent joint [101,102]. Ideally, a TPO should be performed in dogs less than 10 months of age. A TPO is contraindicated once OA is present. Whether a TPO is indicated in asymptomatic dogs with radiographic evidence of hip laxity remains controversial; however, many clinicians believe the potential success of conservative medical therapy precludes the use of a TPO unless significant clinical signs are present.

Another surgical procedure recommended for young dogs without evidence of OA is juvenile pubic symphysiodesis (JPS). JPS is a relatively simple surgical procedure used to close the pubic symphysis prematurely. Premature closure of the pubic symphysis results in ventrolateral rotation of the acetabulum, which increases acetabular ventroversion and the acetabular angle to improve coverage of the femoral head [104]. A ventral approach to the pubis is performed, and electrocautery is applied every 2 to 3 mm along the symphysis at 40 W for 12 to 30 seconds [105]. Improvement in hip conformation is greater when the procedure is performed in dogs between 3 and 4 months of age [106]. When JPS was performed in dogs at 15 weeks of age, the acetabular angle was increased by 16°. When JPS was performed in dogs at 20 weeks of age, the increase in acetabular angle was only 8°, however. Dogs older than 6 months of age do not benefit from JPS surgery [107,108]. Few complications are reported with JPS, although narrowing of the pelvic canal does occur.

In dysplastic dogs with OA that are unresponsive to medical therapy, total hip arthroplasty (THA) is recommended [109]. The procedure to implant the prosthetic hip components requires specialized equipment and training but yields excellent results in most cases. Generally, THA is performed after the dog reaches skeletal maturity. If possible, the dysplastic dogs are managed medically until they are at least 10 to 12 months of age before performing THA. Alternatively, femoral head and neck excision (FHNE) arthroplasty can be performed [110,111]. The goal is to eliminate hip pain by removing the femoral head and neck and initiating the development of a fibrous pseudoarthrosis that permits ambulation. The procedure can be performed in dogs of all sizes; however, results are usually better in smaller and lighter dogs (< 20 kg). FHNE arthroplasty is the current surgery of choice for smaller dogs with HD that are unresponsive to medical treatment. FHNE arthroplasty can also be used with success in large dogs.

Prognosis
The prognosis for dogs with HD is variable. With proper medical management, many dogs maintain a good quality of life without surgical intervention. The prognosis after surgical treatment is good with proper patient selection, sound surgical technique, and proper postoperative management.

ELBOW DYSPLASIA
Canine elbow dysplasia (CED) is a term used to describe all developmental conditions resulting in elbow arthrosis, regardless of the underlying cause. Currently, CED is typically used to describe a complex of developmental abnormalities of the elbow, including ununited anconeal process (UAP), fragmented medial cornoid process (FMCP) (Fig. 5), OC of the medial portion of the humeral condyle, and elbow incongruity [112–118].

Signalment
CED typically affects large- and giant-breed dogs that are rapidly growing. CED may also affect medium-sized and chondrodystrophic dogs [114,116,119–121]. No sex predilection has been observed in dogs with UAP and OC. Male dogs are more commonly affected with FMCP [122]. Bilateral joint involvement is common, and the right and left limbs are equally represented.

Etiology and pathogenesis
The etiology and pathogenesis of CED remain poorly understood, although genetics, nutritional excesses or deficiencies, growth disturbances, OC, and trauma are proposed causes. Pathologic mechanisms proposed to explain the

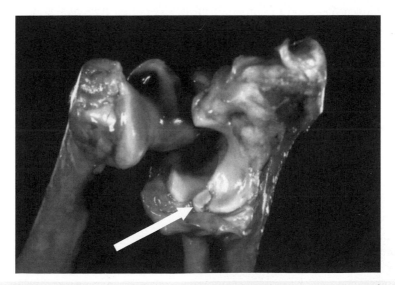

Fig. 5. Elbow specimen (cadaver) from a dog with an FMCP (*arrow*). (Courtesy of Roy R. Pool, DVM, PhD, Texas A&M College of Veterinary Medicine, College Station, Texas.)

development of the primary lesions of CED are OC, trochlear notch dysplasia, and asynchronous growth of the radius and ulna.

Clinical signs

Forelimb lameness is usually present for several months beginning at 4 to 12 months of age. Younger dogs and dogs as old as 8 years of age have been diagnosed, however. The lameness is gradual and progressive and usually worse after exercise. Other signs of CED include short striding and difficulty in rising or lying down. Most dogs with CED sit or stand with the elbow adducted and the carpus abducted. Palpation of the elbows often reveals soft tissue swelling, muscle atrophy, pain, and crepitus. Pain in the elbow is noted on flexion or when the antibrachium is pronated or supinated. A reduced range of motion may also be noted in some dogs.

Diagnosis

A thorough physical examination with lameness evaluation at a walk, trot, and circling figure-of-eight pattern should be performed. Although dogs normally place 60% of their body weight on their forelimbs, dogs with CED often place only 40% to 50%. Both elbows are radiographed to identify bilateral disease and to allow comparison between joints. Several radiographic views are recommended, including a craniocaudal, mediolateral, flexed mediolateral, and craniocaudal medial-to-lateral oblique with the elbow maximally extended and supinated 15°; a mediodistal-to-lateroproximal 30° oblique view is also helpful in some cases [114,123]. Positive-contrast arthrography may be used if OC is suspected to determine the size of subchondral defects, the presence of a radiolucent flap, and the presence of unmineralized free joint bodies [124]. CT and MRI are extremely helpful in the diagnosis of elbow diseases. Nuclear scintigraphy and arthroscopy may also be helpful in confirming the presence of CED.

Fragmented medial coronoid process

Treatment

Medical therapy for FMCP includes weight control, activity restrictions, and medications for pain and OA. Surgical treatment involves the removal of loose or free-floating cartilage or bone fragments and correction of articular incongruence [124,125]. Surgery is performed by medial elbow arthrotomy or arthroscopy (Fig. 6). In most cases, surgery is recommended for dogs with clinical or radiographic signs of FMCP that are less than 12 months of age and for older dogs with large lesions [126]. Dogs with severe radiographic signs of OA may be poor candidates for surgery and are often managed conservatively. Two published studies found that surgical intervention had little advantage over conservative medial therapy in dogs with FMCP [127,128]. Many surgeons find that clinical function improves after surgical removal of the fragmented coronoid process, however, although lameness and pain often recur as OA progresses.

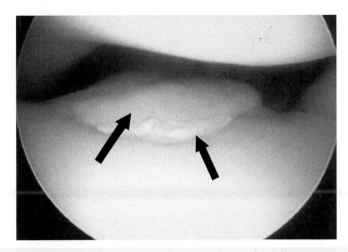

Fig. 6. Arthroscopic view of the craniomedial compartment of the elbow joint in a dog with an FMCP. Arrows identify the FMCP.

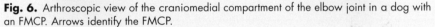

Prognosis

The prognosis for dogs with FMCP varies and may depend primarily on the severity of clinical signs, progression of OA, and treatment used. Early diagnosis and treatment with surgery may provide the best clinical outcome. The increasing use of arthroscopy may also improve the prognosis in those patients undergoing surgery. Surgery is not curative, however, and secondary OA often develops, necessitating chronic medical therapy to control pain and lameness. Factors that do not seem to affect long-term outcome prognosis include the dog's age at the time of surgery and the surgical approach used [129].

Ununited anconeal process

Treatment

Although the condition varies among breeds, the anconeal process remains ununited if it is not attached by 20 weeks of age (Fig. 7). Surgery is recommended for treatment of UAP. Surgical options include removal of the UAP, surgical reattachment, and osteotomy or ostectomy of the ulna with or without surgical fixation of the anconeal process [113,114,130]. Medical management alone is usually less successful than surgery, resulting in rapid progression of OA [131]. Surgical reattachment using a lag screw is usually attempted before 24 weeks of age. After 24 weeks of age, surgical removal of the UAP is usually recommended. Removal of the UAP may also be warranted after osteotomy of the ulna if fusion does not occur within 12 to 18 weeks after surgery.

Prognosis

Long-term evaluations have found that dogs treated with excision of the UAP have a favorable prognosis. A study of 10 dogs in which the UAP was

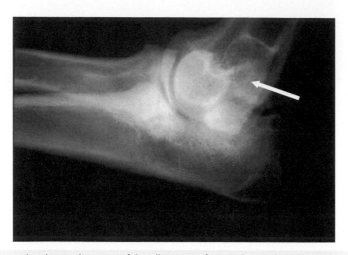

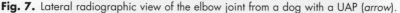

Fig. 7. Lateral radiographic view of the elbow joint from a dog with a UAP (*arrow*).

surgically reattached found encouraging results, though long-term studies are still needed [132]. Osteotomy of the ulna with or without lag screw fixation has produced good clinical outcomes in the long-term studies, but 30% of the patients developed signs of progressive OA [133].

Osteochondrosis dissecans
Treatment
Medical therapy is used primarily for small lesions and consists of rest, weight control, and medication consisting of NSAIDS and OA disease–modifying drugs. Surgery is typically performed by medial arthrotomy or arthroscopy. Arthroscopy provides a less invasive alternative to arthrotomy and is the preferred method of treatment [134,135].

Prognosis
The prognosis after medical or surgical treatment of elbow OCD is guarded. Progression of OA is common and may require chronic medical therapy to control clinical signs. Early surgical treatment of the OCD lesion often decreases lameness but may not prevent the progression of OA.

Elbow incongruity
Treatment
Elbow incongruity is likely caused by asynchronous growth of the radius and ulna and is treated surgically. Radioulnar bowing and rotation that clinically affect the elbow or carpal joint should be addressed early to avoid dysfunction and the potential for severe OA [13]. Addressing the disease with corrective ulnar or radial ostectomy or osteotomy can provide more synchronous growth and less stress on the elbow joint. In more severe cases, treatment options may

include medical therapy, arthrodesis, elbow replacement, corrective osteotomy, or limb amputation.

Prognosis

The prognosis for elbow incongruity varies and may depend on the patient's age, severity of clinical signs, degree of incongruity, and progression of OA. Early surgical intervention may prevent or reduce angular limb deformities and progression of secondary OA.

PES VARUS

Signalment

Pes varus is characterized by a medial bowing of the distal tibia, resulting in deviation of the tarsus and phalanges toward midline (varus deformity). This DOD has been documented in dachshunds and is seen unilaterally or bilaterally [136].

Etiology and pathogenesis

Although there are no studies to validate the claim, this condition is thought to be genetic. Trauma to the medial distal tibial growth plate may cause a similar deformity, but most dogs presented for pes varus have no history of trauma.

Clinical signs

Muscle atrophy or lameness may be present on the clinically affected leg, or the patient may be asymptomatic despite the deformity.

Diagnosis

Physical examination and a thorough history to rule out trauma are usually sufficient to make this diagnosis. Radiographic evidence includes shortening of the medial aspect of the tibia in relation to the lateral cortex and thus a medial bowing of the distal tibia. Osteophyte formation can also be seen on the cranial aspect of the distal tibia [136].

Treatment

Clinical signs of lameness and muscle atrophy should be used to dictate the need for surgical intervention. An open wedge osteotomy and external fixation have been used [137].

Prognosis

Surgical intervention yields excellent results, and dogs without clinical signs do not seem to develop OA of the talocrural joint [137].

SUMMARY

DODs are a common cause of pain and lameness in dogs. Although the etiology of these diseases is not always known, the clinical and radiographic findings associated with each disease are well documented. A thorough history and careful physical examination often help to localize the abnormality; however, radiographic evaluation is usually required to confirm the diagnosis. Treatment varies depending on the type of developmental disease present.

References
[1] Lenehan TM, Fetter AW. Hypertrophic osteodystrophy. In: Newton CD, Nunamaker DM, editors. Textbook of small animal orthopaedics. Philadelphia: JB Lippincott; 1985. p. 597–601.
[2] Alexander JW. Selected skeletal dysplasia: craniomandibular osteopathy, multiple cartilaginous exostosis, and hypertrophic osteodystrophy. Vet Clin North Am Small Anim Pract 1982;13(1):55–70.
[3] Muir P, Dubielzig RR, Johnson KA, et al. Hypertrophic osteodystrophy and calvarial hyperostosis. Compend Contin Educ Pract Vet 1996;18:143–51.
[4] Watson ADJ, Blair RC, Farrow BRH, et al. Hypertrophic osteodystrophy in the dog. Aust Vet J 1973;49(9):433–9.
[5] Bohning R, Suter P, Hohn RB, et al. Clinical and radiographic survey of canine panosteitis. J Am Vet Med Assoc 1970;156:870–84.
[6] Alexander JW. Hypertrophic osteodystrophy. Canine Pract 1978;5:48–52.
[7] Grondalen J. Metaphyseal osteopathy (hypertrophic osteodystrophy) in growing dogs: a clinical study. J Small Anim Pract 1976;17(11):721–35.
[8] Munjar TA, Austin CC, Breur GJ. Comparison of risk factors for hypertrophic osteodystrophy, craniomandibular osteopathy, and canine distemper virus infection. Vet Comp Orthop Traumatol 1998;11:37–43.
[9] Bohning R, Suter P, Hohn RB, et al. Clinical and radiographic survey of canine panosteitis. J Am Vet Med Assoc 1970;156:870–84.
[10] Bellah JR. Hypertrophic osteodystrophy. In: Bojrab MJ, editor. Disease mechanisms in small animal surgery. 2nd edition. Philadelphia: WB Saunders; 1993. p. 859–64.
[11] Woodard JC. Canine hypertrophic osteodystrophy: a study of the spontaneous disease littermates. Vet Pathol 1982;19:337–54.
[12] Holmes JR. Suspected skeletal scurvy in the dog. Vet Rec 1962;74:801–13.
[13] Cook JL. Forelimb lameness in the young patient. Vet Clin North Am Small Anim Pract 2001;31:55–83.
[14] Newton CD, Biery DN. Skeletal diseases. In: Ettinger SJ, editor. Textbook of veterinary internal medicine. 3rd edition. Philadelphia: WB Saunders; 1989. p. 2391–2.
[15] Johnston SA. Joint and skeletal diseases. In: Leib MS, Monroa WE, editors. Practical small animal internal medicine. Philadelphia: WB Saunders; 1997. p. 1189–208.
[16] Schulz KS, Payne JT, Aronson E. Escherichia coli bacteremia associated with hypertrophic osteodystrophy in a dog. J Am Vet Med Assoc 1991;199:1170–3.
[17] Abeles V, Harrus S, Angles JM, et al. Hypertrophic osteodystrophy in six weimaraner puppies associated with systemic signs. Vet Rec 1999;145:130–4.
[18] Harrus S, Waner T, Aizenberg I, et al. Development of hypertrophic osteodystrophy and antibody response in a litter of vaccinated weimaraner puppies. J Small Anim Pract 2002;43:27–31.
[19] Burt JK, Wilson GP. A study of eosinophilic panosteitis (enostosis) in German shepherd dogs. Acta Radiol 1972;319:7–13.
[20] Hulse DA, Johnson AL. Other diseases of bones and joints. In: Small animal surgery. St. Louis: Mosby-Year Book; 1997. p. 1009–30.
[21] Milton JL. Panosteitis: a review of the literature and 32 cases. Auburn Vet 1979;35(3): 11–5.
[22] Lenehan TM, Van Sickle DC, Biery DN. Canine panosteitis. In: Fossum TW, editor. Textbook of small animal orthopaedics. Philadelphia: JB Lippincott; 1985. p. 591–6.
[23] McLaughlin RM. Hind limb lameness in the young patient. Vet Clin North Am Small Anim Pract 2001;31:101–23.
[24] Barrett RB, Schall WD, Lewis RE. Clinical and radiographic features of canine panosteitis. J Am Anim Hosp Assoc 1968;4(2):94–104.
[25] Muir P, Dubielzig RR, Johnson KA. Panosteitis. Compend Contin Educ Pract Vet 1996;18: 29–33.

[26] Craig PH, Riser WH. Osteochondritis dissecans in the proximal humerus of the dog. J Am Vet Radiol Soc 1965;6:40.

[27] Rudd RG, Whitehair JC, Margolis JH. Results of management of osteochondritis dissecans of the humeral head in dogs: 44 cases (1982–1987). J Am Anim Hosp Assoc 1990;26:173–8.

[28] Cordy DR, Wind AP. Transverse fracture of the proximal humeral articular cartilage in dogs. Pathol Vet 1969;6:424–36.

[29] Van Ryssen B, van Bree H, Missinne S. Successful arthroscopic treatment of shoulder osteochondrosis in the dog. J Small Anim Pract 1993;34:521–8.

[30] Vaughan LC, Jones DGC. Osteochondrosis dissecans of the head of a humerus in dogs. J Small Anim Pract 1990;9:283–94.

[31] Probst CW, Flo GL. Comparison of two caudolateral approaches to the scapulohumeral joint for treatment of dissecans in dogs. J Am Vet Med Assoc 1987;191:1101.

[32] Peterson CJ. Osteochondrosis dissecans of the humeral head of a cat. N Z Vet J 1984;32:115.

[33] LaHue TR, Brown SG, Rouch JC, et al. entrapment of joint mice in the bicipital tendon sheath as a sequela to osteochondrosis dissecans of the proximal humerus in dogs: A report of 6 cases. J Am Anim Hosp Assoc 1988;24(1):99–105.

[34] Olsson SE, Reiland S. The nature of osteochondrosis in animals. Acta Radiol Suppl 1978;358:299–306.

[35] Clanton CS, Hilley HD, Henrickson CK, et al. The ultrastructure of osteochondrosis of the articular-epiphyseal complex in growing swine. Calcif Tissue Int 1986;38:44.

[36] Siffert RS. Classification of osteochondroses. Clin Orthop 1981;158:10–8.

[37] Milton JL. Osteochondrosis dissecans in the dog. Vet Clin North Am Small Anim Pract 1983;13(1):117–34.

[38] Johnson AL, Pijanowski GJ, Stein LE. Osteochondritis dissecans of the femoral head of a Pekingese. J Am Vet Med Assoc 1982;187(6):623–5.

[39] Whitehair JG, Rudd RG. Osteochondrosis dissecans of the humeral head in dogs. Compend Contin Educ Pract Vet 1990;12(2):195–204.

[40] Brinker WO, Piermattei DL, Flo GL. Diagnosis and treatment of orthopedic conditions of the forelimb. In: Brinker, Piermattei, and Flo's handbook of small animal orthopedics and fracture treatment. 2nd edition. Philadelphia: WB Saunders; 1990. p. 486–9.

[41] Olsson SE. The early diagnosis of fragmented coronoid process and osteochondritis dissecans of the canine joint. J Am Anim Hosp Assoc 1983;19(5):616–25.

[42] Grondalen J. Arthrosis with special reference to the elbow joint in rapidly rowing dogs. II. Occurrence, clinical and radiographic findings. Nord Vet Med 1979;31(1):69–75.

[43] Goring RL, Bloomberg MS. Selected developmental abnormalities of the canine elbow: Radiographic evaluation and surgical management. Compend Contin Educ Pract Vet 1983;5(3):178–88.

[44] Piermattei DL, Flo GL. The elbow joint. In: Brinker, Piermattei, and Flo's handbook of small animal orthopedics and fracture repair. 3rd edition. Philadelphia: WB Saunders; 1997. p. 288–320.

[45] Montgomery RD, Milton JL, Henderson RA, et al. Osteochondrosis dissecans of the canine stifle. Compend Contin Educ Pract Vet 1989;11(10):1199–205.

[46] Denny HR, Gibbs C. Osteochondritis dissecans of the canine stifle joint. J Small Anim Pract 1980;21(6):317–22.

[47] Leighton RL. Surgical treatment of osteochondritis dissecans of the canine stifle. Vet Med Small Animal Clin 1981;76(12):1733–6.

[48] Beale BS, Goring RL, Herrington J, et al. A prospective evaluation of four surgical approaches to the talus of the dog used in the treatment of osteochondritis dissecans. J Am Anim Hosp Assoc 1991;27:221–9.

[49] Fitch RB, Beale BS. Osteochondrosis of the canine tarsal joint. Vet Clin North Am Small Anim Pract 1998;28(1):95–113.

[50] Probst CW, Johnston SA. Osteochondrosis. In: Slatter DH, editor. Textbook of small animal surgery. Philadelphia: WB Saunders; 1993. p. 1944–66.

[51] Montgomery RD, Hathcock JT, Milton JL, et al. Osteochondritis dissecans of the canine tarsal joint. Compend Contin Educ Pract Vet 1994;16:835–44.

[52] Wisner ER, Berry CR, Morgan JP, et al. Osteochondrosis of the lateral trochlear ridge of the talus in seven rottweiler dogs. Vet Surg 1990;19:435–9.

[53] Rosenblum GP, Robins GM, Carlisle CH. Osteochondritis dissecans of the tibio-tarsal joint in the dog. J Small Anim Pract 1978;19(12):759–67.

[54] Carlisle CH, Robins GM, Reynolds KM. Radiographic signs of osteochondritis dissecans of the lateral ridge of the trochlear tali in the dog. J Small Anim Pract 1990; 31:280–6.

[55] Richardson DC, Zenrek J. Nutrition and osteochondrosis. Vet Clin North Am Small Anim Pract 1998;28:115–35.

[56] Olsson SE. Pathophysiology, morphology, and clinical signs of osteochondrosis in the dog. In: Bojrab MJ, editor. Disease mechanisms in small animal surgery. 2nd edition. Philadelphia: Lippincott Williams & Wilkins; 1993. p. 777–96.

[57] Person MW. Arthroscopy of the canine shoulder joint. Compend Contin Educ Pract Vet 1986;8:537–46.

[58] Van Ryssen B, van Bree H, Vyt Ph. Arthroscopy of the shoulder joint in the dog. J Am Anim Hosp Assoc 1993;29:101–5.

[59] Piermattei DL, Flo GL. Arthrology. In: Brinker, Piermattei, and Flo's handbook of small animal orthopedics and fracture repair. 3rd edition. Philadelphia: WB Saunders; 1997. p. 170–200.

[60] Van Ryssen B, van Bree H. Elbow arthroscopy in the diagnosis of fragmented cornoid process (FCP) in the dog. In: Arthroscopy in the treatment and diagnosis of osteochondrosis in the dog [doctoral dissertation]. Ghent: University of Ghent; 1996. p. 37.

[61] Piermattei DL. The hindlimb. In: Piermattei DL, Johnson KA, editors. An atlas of surgical approaches to the bones and joints of the dog and cat. 3rd edition. Philadelphia: WB Saunders; 1993. p. 276–87.

[62] McLaughlin RM, Hurtig RM, Fries CL. Operative arthroscopy in the treatment of bilateral stifle osteochondritis dissecans in the dog. Vet Comp Orthop Traumatol 1989;4: 158–61.

[63] Miller CW, Presnell KR. Examination of the canine stifle: arthroscopic versus arthrotomy. J Am Anim Hosp Assoc 1985;21:623–9.

[64] Bertrand SG, Lewis DD, Madison JB, et al. Arthroscopic examination and treatment of osteochondritis dissecans of the femoral condyle of six dogs. J Am Anim Hosp Assoc 1997;33:451–5.

[65] Smith MM, Vasseur PB, Morgan MP, et al. Clinical evaluation of dogs affected after surgical and nonsurgical management of osteochondritis dissecans of the talus. J Am Vet Med Assoc 1985;187(1):31–5.

[66] Van Ryssen B, van Bree H. Arthroscopic evaluation of osteochondrosis lesions in the canine hock: a review of two cases. J Am Anim Hosp Assoc 1992;28:295–9.

[67] Van Ryssen B, van Bree H. Arthroscopic evaluation of osteochondrosis lesions in the canine hock joint. J Am Anim Hosp Assoc 1992;28:295–9.

[68] Cook JL, Tomlinson JL, Stoll MR, et al. Arthroscopic removal and curettage of osteochondrosis lesions on the lateral and medial trochlear ridges of the talus in two dogs. J Am Anim Hosp Assoc 2001;37:75–80.

[69] Breur GJ, Spaulding HA, Braden TD. Osteochondritis dissecans of the medial trochlear ridge of the talus in a dog. Vet Comp Orthop Traumatol 1989;4:168–76.

[70] Warren DV, Dingwall JS. Legg-Perthes disease in the dog: a review. Can Vet J 1972;13(6): 135–7.

[71] Nunamaker DM. Legg-Calvé-Perthes disease. In: Newton CD, Nunamaker DM, editors. Textbook of small animal orthopaedics. Philadelphia: JB Lippincott; 1985. p. 949–52.

[72] Lee R, Fry PD. Some observations on the occurrence of Legg-Calvé-Perthes disease (coxa plana) in the dog, and an evaluation of excision arthroplasty as a method of treatment. J Small Anim Pract 1969;10(5):309–17.

[73] Junggren GL. A comparative study of conservative and surgical treatment of Legg Perthes disease in the dog. J Am Anim Hosp Assoc 1966;1:6–10.

[74] Gambardella PC. Legg-Calvé-Perthes disease in dogs. In: Bojrab MJ, editor. Disease mechanisms in small animal surgery. 2nd edition. Philadelphia: Lippincott Williams & Wilkins; 1993. p. 804–7.

[75] Vasseur PB, Foley P, Stevenson S, et al. Mode of inheritance of Perthes disease in Manchester terriers. Clin Orthop 1989;244:281–92.

[76] Ljunggren G. Legg-Perthes disease in the dog. Acta Orthop Scand 1967;95:7–79.

[77] Gibson KL, Lewis DD, Pechman RD. Use of external coaptation for the treatment of avascular necrosis of the femoral head in a dog. J Am Vet Med Assoc 1990;197(7): 868–70.

[78] Lust G, Williams AJ, Burton-Wurster N, et al. Joint laxity and its association with hip dysplasia in Labrador Retrievers. Am J Vet Res 1993;54:1990–9.

[79] Lust G, Geary JC, Sheffy BE. Development of hip dysplasia in dogs. Am J Vet Res 1973;34: 87–91.

[80] Riser WH. Canine hip dysplasia: cause and control. J Am Vet Med Assoc 1974;165:360–2.

[81] Douglas SW, Williamson HD. Veterinary radiological interpretation. Philadelphia: Lea & Febiger; 1970.

[82] Corley EA. Role of the Orthopedic Foundation for Animals in the control of canine hip dysplasia. Vet Clin North Am 1992;22:579–93.

[83] Corley EA, Hogan PM. Trends in hip dysplasia control: analysis of radiographs submitted to the Orthopedic Foundation for Animals, 1974–1984. J Am Vet Med Assoc 1985;187: 805–9.

[84] Heyman SJ, Smith GK, Cofone MA. Biomechanical study of the effect of coxofemoral positioning on passive hip joint laxity in dogs. Am J Vet Res 1993;54:210–5.

[85] Smith GK, Biery DN, Gregor TP. New concepts of coxofemoral joint stability and the development of a clinical stress-radiographic method for quantitating hip joint laxity in the dog. J Am Vet Med Assoc 1990;196:59–70.

[86] Smith GK, Gregor TP, Rhodes WH, et al. Coxofemoral joint laxity from distraction radiography and its contemporaneous and prospective correlation with laxity, subjective score, and evidence of degenerative joint disease from conventional hip-extended radiography in dogs. Am J Vet Res 1993;54:1021–42.

[87] Farese JP, Lust G, Williams AJ, et al. Comparison of measurements of dorsolateral subluxation of the femoral head and maximal passive laxity for evaluation of the coxofemoral joint in dogs. Am J Vet Res 1999;60:1571–6.

[88] Farese JP, Todhunter RJ, Lust G, et al. Dorsolateral subluxation of hip joints in dogs measured in a weight-bearing position with radiography and computed tomography. Vet Surg 1998;27:393–405.

[89] Budsberg SC, Johnston SA, Schwarz PD, et al. Efficacy of etodolac for the treatment of osteoarthritis of the hip joints in dogs. J Am Vet Med Assoc 1999;214:206–10.

[90] Canapp SO, McLaughlin RM, Hoskinson JJ, et al. Scintigraphic evaluation of glucosamine hydrochloride and chondroitin sulfate as treatments for acute synovitis in dogs. Am J Vet Res 1999;60:1550–6.

[91] De Haan JJ, Goring R, Beale BS. Evaluation of polysulfated glycosaminoglycan for the treatment of hip dysplasia in dogs. Vet Surg 1994;23:177–81.

[92] Fox SM, Johnston SA. Use of carprofen for the treatment of pain and inflammation in dogs. J Am Vet Med Assoc 1997;210:1493–8.

[93] Johnston SA, Budsberg SC. Nonsteroidal anti-inflammatory drugs and corticosteroids for the management of canine osteoarthritis. Vet Clin North Am Small Anim Pract 1997;27: 841–62.

[94] Johnston SA, Fox SM. Mechanisms of actions of anti-inflammatory medications used for the treatment of osteoarthritis. J Am Vet Med Assoc 1997;210:1486–92.

[95] Lippiello L, Idouraine A, McNamara PS, et al. Cartilage stimulatory and antiproteolytic activity is present in sera of dogs treated with a chondroprotective agent. Canine Pract 1999;24:18–9.

[96] Lust G, Williams MS, Burton-Wurster N, et al. Effects of intramuscular administration of glycosaminoglycan polysulfates on signs of incipient hip dysplasia in growing pups. Am J Vet Res 1992;53:1836–43.

[97] McNamara PS, Johnston SA, Todhunter RJ. Slow-acting, disease-modifying osteoarthritis agents. Vet Clin North Am Small Anim Pract 1997;27:841–62.

[98] Millis DL, Levine D. The role of exercise and physical modalities in the treatment of osteoarthritis. Vet Clin North Am Small Anim Pract 1997;27:841–62.

[99] Vasseur PB, Johnson AL, Budsberg SC, et al. Randomized, controlled trial of the efficacy of carprofen, a nonsteroidal anti-inflammatory drug, on the treatment of osteoarthritis in dogs. J Am Vet Med Assoc 1995;206:807–11.

[100] Hosgood G, Lewis DD. Retrospective evaluation of fixation complications of 49 pelvic osteotomies in 36 dogs. J Small Anim Pract 1993;34:123–30.

[101] McLaughlin RM, Miller CW. Evaluation of hip joint congruence and range of motion before and after triple pelvic osteotomy. Vet Comp Orthop Traumatol 1991;4:65–9.

[102] McLaughlin RM, Miller CW, Taves CL, et al. Force plate analysis of triple pelvic osteotomy for the treatment of canine hip dysplasia. Vet Surg 1991;20:291–7.

[103] Slocum B, Devine T. Pelvic osteotomy technique for axial rotation of the acetabular segment in dogs. J Am Anim Hosp Assoc 1986;22:331–8.

[104] Mathews KG, Stover SM, Kass PH. Effect of pubis symphysiodesis on acetabular and pelvic development in guinea pigs. Am J Vet Res 1996;57:1427–33.

[105] Patricell AJ, Dueland RT, Yan L, et al. Canine pubic symphysiodesis: investigation of electrocautery dose response by histologic examination and temperature measurement. Vet Surg 2001;30:261–8.

[106] Swainson SW, Conzemius MG, Riedesel EA, et al. Effect of pubic symphysiodesis on pelvic development in the skeletally immature greyhound. Vet Surg 2001;29:178–90.

[107] Dueland RT, Adams WM, Fialowski JP, et al. Effects of symphysiodesis in dysplastic puppies. Vet Surg 2001;30:201–17.

[108] Patricelli AJ, Dueland RT, Adams WM, et al. Juvenile pubic symphysiodesis in dysplastic puppies at 15 and 20 weeks of age. Vet Surg 2002;31:435–44.

[109] Olmstead ML, Hohn RB, Turner TM. A five-year study of 221 total hip replacements in the dog. J Am Vet Med Assoc 1983;183:191–4.

[110] Berzon JL, Howard PE, Covell SJ, et al. A retrospective study of the efficacy of femoral head and neck excisions in 94 dogs and cats. Vet Surg 1980;9:88–92.

[111] Gendreau C, Cawley AJ. Excision of the femoral head and neck: the long-term results of 35 operations. J Am Anim Hosp Assoc 1977;13:605–8.

[112] Elbow database. Columbia, MO: Orthopedic Foundation for Animals; 2001.

[113] Fox SM, Bloomberg MS, Bright RM. Developmental anomalies of the canine elbow. J Am Anim Hosp Assoc 1983;19:605–15.

[114] Goring RL, Bloomberg MS. Selected developmental abnormalities of the canine elbow: radiographic evaluation and surgical management. Compend Contin Educ Pract Vet 1983;5:178–88.

[115] Piermattei DL, Flo GL. The elbow joint. In: Brinker WO, Piermattei DL, Flo GL, editors. Brinker, Piermattei, and Flo's handbook of small animal orthopedics and fracture repair. 3rd edition. Philadelphia: WB Saunders; 1997. p. 288–320.

[116] Stevens DR, Sande RD. An elbow dysplasia syndrome in the dog. J Am Vet Med Assoc 1974;165:1065–9.

[117] Zontine WJ, Weitkamp RA, Lippincott CL. Redefined type of elbow dysplasia involving calcified flexor tendons attached to the medial humeral epicondyle in three dogs. J Am Vet Med Assoc 1989;194:1082–5.

[118] Kirberger RM, Fourie SL. Elbow dysplasia in the dog: pathophysiology, diagnosis and control. J S Afr Vet Assoc 1998;69(2):43–54.

[119] Wind AP. Elbow incongruity and developmental elbow diseases in the dog. Part I. J Am Anim Hosp Assoc 1986;22:711–24.

[120] Ljunggren G, Cawley AJ, Archibald J. The elbow dysplasias in the dog. J Am Vet Med Assoc 1966;148:887–91.

[121] Hare WCD. Congenital detachment of the processus anconeus in the dog. Vet Rec 1956;74:545–6.

[122] Schwarz PD. Canine elbow dysplasia. In: Bonagura JD, editor. Kirk's current veterinary therapy XIII. Philadelphia: WB Saunders; 2000. p. 1004–14.

[123] Marcellin-Little DJ, Stebbins ME, Haudiquet P. The mediodistal to lateroproximal oblique (MEDLAP) radiographic view enhances visualization of the medial coronoid process in dogs. Presented at the 11th Annual American College of Veterinary Surgeons Veterinary Symposium. Washington, DC; 2001.

[124] Lewis DD, Parker RB, Hager DA. Fragmented medial coronoid process of the canine elbow. Compend Contin Educ Pract Vet 1989;11(6):703–34.

[125] Boulay JP. Fragmented coronoid process of the ulna of the dog. Vet Clin North Am Small Anim Pract 1998;28:51–74.

[126] Lewis DD, McCarthy RJ, Pechman RD. Diagnosis of common developmental orthopedic conditions in canine pediatric patients. Compend Contin Educ Pract Vet 1992;14(3):287–301.

[127] Bouck GR, Miller CW, Taves CL. A comparison of surgical and medical treatment of fragmented coronoid process and osteochondritis dissecans of the canine elbow. Vet Comp Orthop Traumatol 1995;8:177–83.

[128] Huibregtse ME, Johnson AL, Muhlbauer MC, et al. The effect of treatment of fragmented coronoid process on the development of osteoarthritis of the elbow. J Am Anim Hosp Assoc 1994;30:190–5.

[129] Tobias TA, Miyabayashi T, Olmstead ML, et al. Surgical removal of fragmented coronoid process in the dog: comparative effects of surgical approach and age at time of surgery. J Am Anim Hosp Assoc 1994;30:360–8.

[130] Sjostrom L, Kasstrom H, Kallberg M. Ununited anconeal process in the dog. Pathogenesis and treatment by osteotomy of the ulna. Vet Comp Orthop Traumatol 1995;8:170–6.

[131] Cross AR, Chambers JN. Ununited anconeal process of the canine elbow. Compend Contin Educ Pract Vet 1997;19(3):349–61.

[132] Fox SM, Burbidge HM, Bray JC, et al. Ununited anconeal process: lag-screw fixation. J Am Anim Hosp Assoc 1996;32:52–6.

[133] Meyer-Lindenberg A, Fehr M, Nolte I. Short- and long-term results after surgical treatment of an ununited anconeal process in the dog. Vet Comp Orthop Traumatol 2001;14:101–10.

[134] Van Bree H, Van Ryssen B. Diagnostic and surgical arthroscopy in osteochondrosis lesions. Vet Clin North Am Small Anim Pract 1998;28:161–89.

[135] Van Ryssen B, van Bree H. Arthroscopic findings in 100 dogs with elbow lameness. Vet Rec 1997;140:360–2.

[136] Mayrhofer E. Metaphysare tibiadysplasie beim dachshund. Kleintierpraxis 1977;22:223–8.

[137] Johnson SG, Hulse DA, Vangundy TE, et al. Corrective osteotomy for pes varus in the dachshund. Vet Surg 1989;18(5):373–9.

Vet Clin Small Anim 35 (2005) 1137–1154

VETERINARY CLINICS
SMALL ANIMAL PRACTICE

Management of Fractures in Small Animals

James K. Roush, DVM, MS

Department of Clinical Sciences, College of Veterinary Medicine, Kansas State University, Manhattan, KS 66506, USA

Fracture repair in small animals has arrived at a crossroads because of advances in fracture repair and client demands. Research into bone healing and repair techniques, collective professional experience, economics, and client demands are obligating veterinarians to greater expertise in the actual act of repairing fractures. These demands leave fewer and fewer general small animal practitioners the time and economic incentive to maintain all-encompassing knowledge about fracture repair. The influx of surgery specialists into burgeoning private practices has improved access to specialty service beyond what the limited number of academic practices could previously provide and has raised the local standard of practice for orthopedic surgery at the same time. Despite ever-increasing referral of small animal orthopedic cases from the general small animal practitioner to specialists, however, the necessity to deal with the preoperative and postoperative management of traumatized small animals by the general practitioner has not changed. Treatment of the small animal patient with a fractured bone does involve accurate definition of the fracture, selection of an appropriate method of fracture fixation from the variety of devices available, and correct application of the fixation. Far more than these, however, it involves assessment and treatment of the traumatized patient as a whole, including preanesthetic evaluation of critical body systems, preoperative preparation of the patient and client, and postoperative management of the repaired fracture and patient.

PREOPERATIVE PATIENT ASSESSMENT

Fractured long bones are often the most obvious effect of trauma but are not the most immediately critical of the possible injuries and are rarely or never life-threatening emergencies. The first and most important actions in fracture diagnosis and management are to (1) thoroughly assess the traumatized animal for other injuries of core body systems, particularly occult injuries to the thorax

---

E-mail address: roushjk@vet.ksu.edu

0195-5616/05/$ – see front matter
doi:10.1016/j.cvsm.2005.06.001

and abdomen; (2) eliminate or stabilize life-threatening injuries to the animal; and (3) provide immediate relief for pain and discomfort from the injuries.

Approximately 60% of animals with limb fractures have radiographic, electrocardiographic, or other evidence of thoracic trauma, whereas only 20% of affected dogs have associated clinical signs [1]. Knowledge of this fact demands that we pay careful attention to the respiratory and cardiovascular systems, regardless of whether the long bone trauma is in the forelimb or hind limb or whether the owner relates a head-on vehicular accident or a glancing blow. It is now accepted standard of care that every animal sustaining vehicular or other trauma sufficient to result in long bone fracture should have routine chest radiographs taken and an electrocardiogram (ECG) performed and scrutinized. Traditionally, chest radiographs would be assessed for the presence of diaphragmatic hernia, but these radiographs should also be carefully evaluated for rib fractures, pneumothorax, hemothorax, pneumomediastinum, pulmonary contusions, traumatic pulmonary bullae, and other trauma that may affect anesthetic protocols and patient survival.

None of these are routinely fatal if properly treated or misdiagnosed. Rib fractures may cause pain during respiration and result in hypoventilation but generally heal with rest and time. The position of rib fragments should be carefully assessed for possible displacement into the pleural cavity, which can result in lung laceration and contribute to pneumothorax or hemothorax. Segmental rib fractures sufficient to creat a "flail" segment of the chest wall are best treated with rest and splints according to recent reports [2]. The diagnosis of pneumothorax should be followed immediately by needle aspiration of the pleural cavity. If negative pressure cannot be achieved through simple aspiration, placement of chest tubes should occur immediately and periodic aspiration or continuous suction should be applied to the tubes. Nasal oxygen supplementation is beneficial in many trauma patients not only to improve Po_2 in circulation and ease respiratory effort but to speed healing of possible myocardial contusions. Cardiac arrhythmias, some potentially fatal, result from myocardial blunt trauma and may not appear until up to 48 to 72 hours after traumatic myocarditis. ECGs that are initially normal should thus be repeated at 3- to 12-hour intervals until 3 days after the trauma, or, alternatively continuous 24-hour monitoring should be instituted. Non–life-threatening cardiac arrhythmias, primarily those that still provide acceptable systolic pressures with each heartbeat and those that are periodic and intermixed with normal contractions, need not be treated beyond oxygen supplementation. Ventricular tachycardia, multifocal premature ventricular contractions, or other life-threatening arrhythmias should be treated by an intravenous antiarrhythmic bolus and then continual infusion [3]. Pulmonary bullae are not dangerous of themselves, but their presence should be noted before anesthesia so that overinflation and subsequent rupture of the bullae can be avoided.

Other body systems should also be evaluated, but complete confidence in findings may be delayed for hours to days. Blunt rupture of abdominal organs, such as intestine, is difficult to detect on initial physical examination. Abdominal radiographs to evaluate free abdominal gas or diagnostic peritoneal lavage may be useful to identify hollow organ injury. Approximately 40% of dogs with pelvic fractures have urinary tract injury [4]. Defecation and urination should be monitored to evaluate gastrointestinal and urinary function. Urinary bladder ruptures are often not detected until up to 48 hours after the trauma, and diligence must be maintained to detect these injuries. Levels of potassium or creatinine in abdominal paracentesis or lavage fluids double or greater than serum levels indicate urinary system rupture.

The neurologic status for each animal must be assessed to rule out central nervous system injuries and peripheral fracture-associated injuries. Obviously, recumbent animals should be particularly assessed for spinal fracture or dislocation. Neurologic integrity is difficult to detect in recumbent animals, particularly those with multilimb injuries, and reassessment of neural function should be performed periodically during the recovery period. A stable nonambulatory animal with only a single identified limb injury particularly must be re-evaluated for the presence of multiple limb or neurologic injuries. As an example, in a recent case of a right tibial fracture (Figs. 1 and 2),

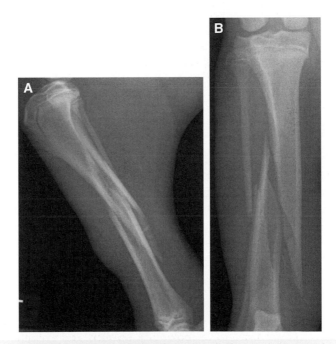

Fig. 1. Lateral (A) and craniocaudal (B) radiographs of a fractured tibia. This fracture would be completely described as a simple, closed, long oblique, diaphyseal fracture of the right tibia displaced laterally and cranially. There is also a simple, closed, short transverse fracture of the midshaft of the right fibula displaced laterally and cranially.

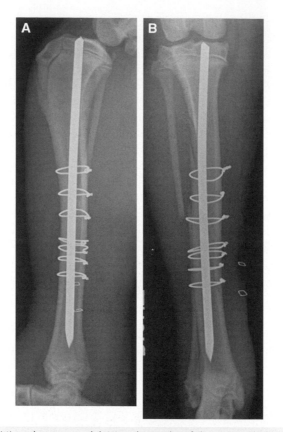

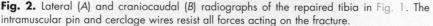

Fig. 2. Lateral (A) and craniocaudal (B) radiographs of the repaired tibia in Fig. 1. The intramuscular pin and cerclage wires resist all forces acting on the fracture.

a recumbent animal with no other detectable abnormalities exhibited a left forelimb proprioceptive deficit (Fig. 3) only after the tibial fracture was repaired and the animal stood without support. The proprioceptive deficit was difficult to detect before surgery in the recumbent animal, and detection was complicated by the owner-supplied history that the dog had walked away from the trauma on three legs (non-weight bearing on the right hind limb).

The long bone fracture itself usually presents with limb dysfunction, pain, fracture instability, overlying soft tissue trauma, abnormal posture or limb position, or crepitus. The veterinarian should carefully evaluate other structures on an affected limb to eliminate "masked" injuries, such as a fractured metacarpal distal to an obviously swollen and crepitant humeral fracture. Fractures below the elbow and knee may be splinted for temporary relief of discomfort, but splints should be removed again for subsequent radiography. The involved limb should be carefully examined for wounds, particularly in the region of the fracture, because open fractures carry an

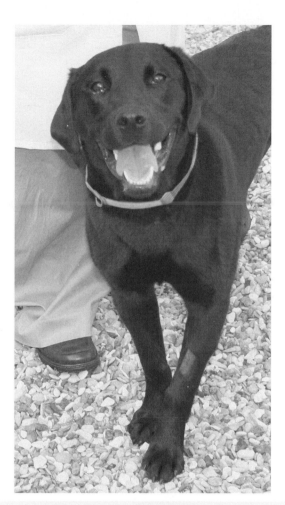

Fig. 3. Proprioceptive deficit on the left front limb discovered after repair of the right tibial fracture.

increased risk of osteomyelitis and other complications and necessitate immediate attention to wound care and cleansing.

All fractures should be radiographed before surgery. Radiography can confirm fracture diagnosis and determine fracture configuration to allow for correct decisions regarding repair of the fracture. At least two divergent views of the entire affected bone (preferably at 90° to one another) are needed to assess fracture configuration accurately and to allow three-dimensional modeling of the fracture. Analgesia or general anesthesia is necessary to provide patient comfort and allow proper positioning of the fractured limb during radiography. Many radiographs in the author's practice are made using acepromazine (0.02 mg/kg administered intravenously) for animal sedation and hydromorphone (0.4 mg/kg administered intravenously) for analgesia, but sedation should be carefully considered in light of the overall condition of the patient. Oblique and skyline radiographic views are often useful in injuries involving multibone joints, such as the carpus and tarsus. Other radiographic modalities, such as CT scans or MRI, are useful for detailing fractures of these joints or of the axial skeleton when available. CT scans, which allow three-dimensional reconstruction, are particularly useful in the surgeon's understanding of pelvic or skull fracture configuration. Bone scintigraphy may be useful to determine the site of bone injury if physical examination does not localize the fracture and may be singularly useful in the diagnosis of nondisplaced fractures and fractures of distal extremity sesamoids.

PAIN MANAGEMENT OF PATIENTS WITH FRACTURE

All patients with fractures deserve adequate pain relief before, during, and after fracture repair. Although some nonsteroidal analgesics, such as deracoxib, are approved for postoperative orthopedic pain in dogs, the author believes that these agents are less than ideal if used for sole analgesia in preoperative and immediate postoperative fracture patients. Most animals with fractures should be given analgesic coverage with narcotic agonists or narcotic agonist-antagonists, such as buprenorphine or butorphanol. Narcotic agonists, such as morphine or hydromorphone, are commonly given, but the required dosage interval of 3 to 4 hours necessitates the availability of 24-hour care to allow proper analgesic coverage overnight. In animals with hind limb fractures, epidurals with narcotic or local anesthetic agents are useful to provide for good pain relief before and after surgery, particularly if indwelling epidural catheters are placed so that repeated administration is convenient. Extradermal narcotic patches containing fentanyl may be used for pain control in dogs or cats before or after surgery. In the author's practice, postoperative patients commonly receive injectable narcotic or oral combination narcotic nonsteroidal anti-inflammatory drugs (NSAIDS), such as acetaminophen-codeine. If fractious, cats may be given buprenorphine orally by squirting the intravenous solution into the mouth, where it is absorbed by the oral mucosa.

TEMPORARY PREOPERATIVE STABILIZATION AND MANAGEMENT

Temporary stabilization of fractures is performed to increase patient comfort, to minimize local soft tissue swelling, and to prevent additional soft tissue injury. Fractures of the lower extremities have less soft tissue coverage and may become open fractures or undergo additional comminution if unsupported. Fractures proximal to the elbow or stifle are difficult to stabilize with external coaptation, and the animal should be cage confined without splinting and treated with analgesics until repair. Fractures distal to the elbow or stifle may be stabilized with external coaptation until repair, particularly during transport to a referral center. Adequate external coaptation for these fractures consists of a Robert-Jones bandage or a modified Robert-Jones bandage incorporating a molded lateral fiberglass splint. Coaptation should immobilize the joint immediately proximal to the fracture and extend distally to the toes.

Open fractures are emergencies in animals. Open fractures should receive immediate cleansing, debridement, and microbial aerobic and anaerobic cultures. Animals should be placed on broad-spectrum antibiotics until culture and sensitivity results are available. The wound should be copiously lavaged with lactated Ringer's solution or another physiologic electrolyte solution. Final stabilization of open fractures at the time of emergency management is not necessary, particularly in hemodynamically unstable animals, but these wounds should be maintained as open wounds under a sterile bandage until surgical stabilization.

PROPHYLACTIC ANTIBIOTIC THERAPY IN FRACTURE PATIENTS

Patients with closed fractures should not be given prophylactic antibiotics over extended periods without a clear indication. Indiscriminate use of systemic broad-spectrum antibiotics is not necessary in clean orthopedic procedures and may lead to an increased risk of nosocomial infection or colonization of the hospital environment with resistant bacteria. Perioperative antibiotics may be beneficial in open surgical procedures that are longer than 2 hours in duration. The author recommends one-time administration of a first-generation cephalosporin at a dose of 20 mg/kg administered intravenously and 20 mg/kg administered intramuscularly (40-mg/kg total dose) to provide prophylactic antibiotic coverage for up to 5 hours of open procedure time. Alternatively, some surgeons prefer to give a dose of cephalosporin (20 mg/kg administered intravenously) and then to follow that with repeat doses at 2-hour intervals until conclusion of the operation. Again, open fracture sites should be cultured and the animal placed on an empiric broad-spectrum antibiotic or antibiotic combination while awaiting culture results.

BONE BIOMECHANICS RELATED TO FRACTURE REPAIR

Bone is viscoelastic and is composed of inorganic (hydroxyapatite) and organic (collagen and cellular) components. Bones undergo elastic and plastic deformation during fracture. The bones of younger animals often deform before breaking, making them hard to reduce adequately, but the plastic phase in older animals may not be evident on examination of the fracture. Bone strength, stiffness, and energy absorption to failure are affected by material properties of the bone, such as composition, morphology, and porosity; by structural components, such as the bone geometry, bone length, and bone curvature; and by other factors, such as the rate, magnitude, and orientation of forces during trauma. Load deformation curves, discussed in many articles on bone biomechanics, are interesting but not useful for fracture repair.

Fractures occur after the application of external or internal forces. Internal forces include those attributable to violent muscle contraction (avulsion fractures) or underlying bone pathologic changes. The configuration of any individual fracture depends on a number of variables occurring at the time of fracture, including the nature, degree, speed of application, and direction of the force(s); the inherent strength and condition of the bone (eg, osteoporosis); and inherent and existing loads on the bone related to body position or muscle contraction. Fracture configuration is influenced by the stored energy in the bone at the time of fracture, and it is particularly influenced by the speed of loading.

A complete understanding of the forces acting on bone is important for good fracture repair. The five forces acting on bone in vivo are bending, compression, shear, tension, and torsion. Bending forces are forces applied to a specific focal point on the bone perpendicular to the long axis of the bone and result in transverse or short oblique fractures of the diaphysis. Compressive forces act along the long axis of the bone and attempt to "shorten" the bone, resulting in impaction of the bone shaft or depression fractures at the articular surface. Shear force is transmitted parallel to but not along the long axis of a bone and results in the fracture of bony prominences along the line of force or in oblique fracture configurations. A Salter IV fracture of the lateral aspect of the humeral condyle in a young dog is a classic shear fracture. Tensile forces act along the long axis of the bone and attempt to "lengthen" the bone, often resulting in transverse fractures of the diaphysis or avulsion fractures at points of muscle origin or insertion. Torsion is a twisting force applied to the long axis of the bone and results in the formation of spiral fracture configurations of the diaphysis. Comminuted fractures are generally the result of multiple loading modes and often result from rapid loading of the bone. Each repair of a fractured bone must allow for and counteract all forces to allow optimal healing.

A final concept to understand, particularly in relation to the use of bone plates, is the concept of functional repair "modes." There are three functional repair modes: compression, neutralization, and buttress. Compression mode occurs when the fracture ends are placed under compression with a dynamic compression plate or a tension jig. Neutralization mode occurs when the fracture fragments are anatomically reconstructed and the plate is placed on the bone so as to neutralize forces across the fracture or, in simpler terms, to transmit the forces "around" the fractured area to protect the repair. Buttress mode plating occurs when there is a gap present in the fracture repair from missing fragments and that gap is bridged by the plate. Buttress plating is prone to plate breakage because of the increased stresses placed on the bone plate if a bone plate is used alone.

BONE HEALING

Bone undergoes healing in three phases similar to those of normal wound repair. The first, the inflammatory phase, lasts several days while the initial hematoma is organized, dead or traumatized cells are removed, and cellular precursors are recruited. As surgeons think of it, bone healing occurs in the reparative phase, where the fracture gap is filled by material resembling bone. The reparative phase lasts approximately 6 to 10 weeks in most dogs. Finally, the remodeling phase occurs when woven bone placed in the fracture gap is replaced by longitudinal haversian systems over time. The remodeling phase lasts essentially for years after fracture until all haversian systems have been completely reformed.

At the time of fracture, the normal intramedullary centrifugal blood supply pattern of bone is disrupted. Most fracture fragments are devascularized, except for specific areas beneath muscle attachments. Bone fragments are revascularized during the reparative phase by formation of a temporary extraosseous blood supply pattern through attachment of surrounding soft tissues to the bone fragments and establishment of a centripetal flow pattern. The normal afferent vascular system returns as the intramedullary blood supply pattern reforms.

Two healing patterns are recognized in bone: primary healing and secondary healing. The type of bone healing is dependent on the strain across the fracture gap. Strain is an important biomechanical term related to the change in the length of the gap when placed under force and is expressed as a percentage of the original gap size. Primary healing occurs when there is direct bridging of the fracture gap by haversian bone. This occurs only under small fracture gaps and under extreme rigidity (<2% strain across the gap). There is a more common form of primary healing, known as gap healing, where woven bone is laid directly into a fracture gap by osteoblasts and then remodeled by haversian bone at a later date; however, again, the strain must be less than 2% across the gap for gap healing to occur. Secondary bone healing occurs when a fracture callus forms. Tissue in the callus initially starts as granulation tissue with lots of pluripotential osteoprogenitor cells present, and the tissue then remodels through phases of fibrous connective tissue, fibrocartilage, and, finally, woven bone as the size and type of the transforming callus decrease the strain across the fracture. Thus, as a general rule, the larger the callus, the greater is the strain the callus is trying to stabilize, with the exception being that the periosteum in young animals is quite sensitive to disturbance, such that exuberant callus forms merely as a result of stripping periosteum off the bone during repair. There is at least one other important fracture healing concept related to strain. In normal fracture healing, if one radiographs a rigidly stable bone repair at approximately 2 weeks, the fracture gap seems to have enlarged. This occurs because bone ends at the fracture are avascular and are re-vascularized and remodeled, enlarging the gap in the process, and thus decreasing the relative strain by increasing the "original" length, improving the environment for direct bone deposition.

FRACTURE DESCRIPTION

A complete, accurate, and conscious description of the fracture should be performed for each fracture. A complete fracture description allows for accurate communication during consultation or referral with a surgical specialist. A complete fracture description with accurate terms provides intuitive insights to proper fracture management. For example, the description of a given fracture as "long oblique" (see Fig. 1) emphasizes to the surgeon that the fracture is perhaps a candidate for the use of cerclage wire as ancillary fixation (see Fig. 2). A complete and systematic description of each fracture minimizes the chances that important components of the fracture are missed. Other systemic factors, such as the animal's age or the presence of underlying bone diseases like osteoporosis, may also affect fracture repair choices and should be taken into account accordingly. Each description of a fracture for the purpose of planning fracture repair should include the bone fractured, fracture location on the bone, fracture configuration, displacement, and presence or absence of environmental contamination. Exact and accurate anatomic terms should be used for the description (Table 1). Fragment displacement is always described from the aspect of where the distal fragment goes in relation to the proximal fragment.

Repaired fractures are often most unstable along the lines of the original fracturing force, because the bone does not aid the implant in fixation along this line. Transverse fractures with no interdigitation are rotationally unstable. Repairing the fracture provides protection against compressive, shear, and bending forces through cortical contact between the fracture ends, but special care must be taken to ensure rotational stability. The most common repair mistake leading to fracture nonunion in veterinary medicine is the sole use of a single intramedullary pin to repair a transverse femur fracture. Advocated as adequate fixation in past decades, it provides no rotational stability and leads to repair failure and fracture nonunion at unacceptable rates for modern fracture repair.

GENERAL PRINCIPLES OF REPAIR

Orthopedic training from the 1950s on has primarily focused on three classic principles of fracture repair: anatomic reduction, rigid stability, and early return to function. On the surface, each of these ideas has been challenged over the past decade, but each remains an important guide even if accepted now in broader terms or under a different guise. In the past, restoration of every fragment to its proper anatomic position was considered supremely important for function. Today, we recognize that the emphasis should be on anatomic positioning of the joint surfaces in relation to the proximal and distal bones for good postoperative function to occur. The "open-but-do-not-touch" (OBDNT) techniques are meant to provide for fracture stability and overall limb alignment but not to reduce individual fragments [5]. The limited surgical approaches of the OBDNT plating techniques preserve blood supply to individual fragments and limit intraoperative contamination, resulting in overall quicker fracture healing and less likelihood of complications. Old techniques, such as that demonstrated in Fig. 2, are still valid methods of repair because they control all forces placed on the fracture even though the same fracture could have been treated with a bone plate or with external skeletal fixation. Newer techniques, such as plate-rod fixation, use old devices in a new pattern to improve fixation of buttress mode fractures (Fig. 4). Likewise, the increasing use of external skeletal or circular fixators also provides for anatomic

Table 1
Descriptive fracture terms

Term	Definition
Proximal	Toward the end of the bone closer to the body axis
Distal	Toward the end of the bone closer to the toes
Metaphyseal	Any fracture within the anatomic metaphysis of a long bone
Diaphyseal	A fracture of the diaphysis of a long bone
Epiphyseal	A fracture involving the epiphysis in a mature animal (with a closed physis); "proximal" or "distal" also applies here
Physeal	A fracture that occurs at or across the physeal line in an immature animal; subdivided into the Salter-Harris (S-H) classification; with each progressive S-H type, there is a poorer prognosis for normal growth and return to function
S-H type I	A complete separation of the epiphysis from the metaphysis along the physis
S-H type II	A fracture that occurs partially along the physis and exits through the metaphysis
S-H type III	A fracture that occurs partially along the physis and exits through the epiphysis
S-H type IV	A fracture that crosses the physis, with one end of the fracture line exiting at metaphysis and the other exiting at the epiphysis
S-H type V	Impaction fracture of the physis
Condylar	A fracture in a mature animal that affects condyles of distal humerus, distal femur, proximal tibia, or talus
Articular	A fracture that involves the articular surface of a bone
Incomplete	A fracture that does not disrupt bone continuity; more definitive terms are depression
	Areas of bone that are allowed to move away from the direction of force by intersection of multiple fissure lines
Fissure	Incomplete fracture composed of cracks that do not form a separate fragment
Greenstick	Incomplete fracture in which one cortex is broken and the opposite cortex is bent; the bent side is usually the compressive side of the fracture
Complete	A fracture that results in loss of bone continuity, allowing overriding and deformation
Simple	The bone is fractured into two separate fragments
Comminuted	Implies at least three fracture fragments with interconnecting fracture lines
Transverse	The fracture line is primarily perpendicular to the long axis of the bone
Oblique	The fracture line angles across the long axis of the bone; the cortices of each fragment are in the same plane rather than spiraling; short oblique fractures are less than twice the bone diameter, and long oblique fractures are greater than twice the bone diameter
Spiral	A fracture line that coils along the long axis of the bone
Impacted	Bone fragments driven firmly together
Avulsion	Site of insertion of a muscle, tendon, or ligament detached as a result of a forceful pull
Segmental	Three or more fracture fragments in a single bone; however, the fracture lines do not interconnect
Multiple	Two or more bones fractured in the same animal
Unicondylar	One condyle is involved or fractured
Bicondylar	Both condyles are involved; common term for "Y" fractures of distal humerus
Eponyms	Certain fractures and diseases are described using a proper name (of the "discoverer"); example: Monteggia's fracture is a cranial luxation of the radial head combined with a proximal third fracture of the ulna

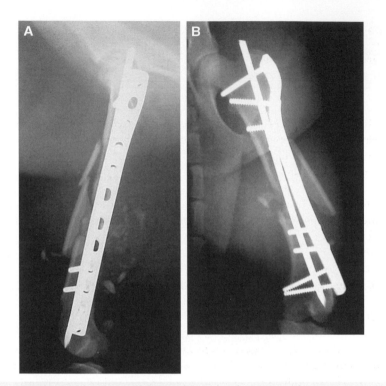

Fig. 4. Lateral (A) and craniocaudal (B) radiographs of a plate-rod fixation combination to repair this comminuted femoral fracture in a dog.

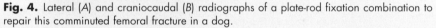

alignment of the bone ends without interfering with the environment at the fracture site. Rigid stability of fixation is still imperative in the early healing of fractures and will remain so because it is based on basic fundamental aspects of bone healing, such as the strain rate under which osteoblasts produce bone instead of cartilage. In later stages of healing, however, ongoing research on staged disassembly or resorbable fracture appliances may show results in improving the speed of bone remodeling or the strength of the bone during the remodeling phase.

The next advancement in orthopedic veterinary care is likely to be in the area of early return to function or, in simpler terms, physical rehabilitation. Early return to function is enhanced by directed physical rehabilitation techniques and results in maintenance of muscular tone and mass in the limb, allows normal joint mobility and joint nutrition, and uses normal weight-bearing forces to maintain bone density in the remainder of the limb.

TO REPAIR OR REFER?

Veterinary medicine as a whole is seeing a rapid increase in the number of private practice specialists of all types. The standard of care for orthopedic surgery has expanded significantly with the influx of specialists into urban private practices and the ease of modern transportation, such that the legal standard is no longer what might have been done in the adjacent county but is, in fact, what would have been done by a board-certified specialist available much closer than in the past. As the local standard of care rises and the distance to specialists decreases, the number of orthopedic procedures performed by general practitioners is likely to decrease. The primary decision is still whether the client and patient would be better served by repair of the fracture locally (convenience, cost, and time benefits) or by referral to a qualified surgeon (better expertise, wider variety of equipment, and more experience), but the equation is tipping toward the latter, because the inconvenience and time of travel to a specialist are decreasing and the economic costs of increased equipment and training to maintain expertise are increasing. Most fracture complications and subsequent problems with client relationships are a direct result of choosing less than adequate methods of repair under pressure from the client regarding procedure costs. Clients who pressure veterinarians into ill-advised repair techniques conveniently (or inconveniently) seem to forget that exchange when fracture complications arise. Cost may be a primary factor in the client choice of local repair versus referral, but unless similar expertise and equipment are available locally, cost should never be the determining factor in a decision not to refer. Fracture complications of malunion, nonunion, or poor limb use inevitably cost more than cost-based compromises save initially [6]. This author firmly believes and teaches that there are almost always acceptable alternative fixation techniques for any given fracture configuration but there are also unacceptable techniques that should not be chosen despite their cost benefit. Most, if not all, complications of fracture repair can be traced to a management or technical error, despite vigorous attempts by the surgeon to ascribe failure to the patient or client. Most often, those unacceptable alternatives can be preemptively identified if analyzing the potential repair for control of each of the five forces acting on the fracture; unacceptable techniques often leave a force or forces unopposed.

REPAIR DECISIONS

There are a number of simple fractures that do not need repair. Fractures of the ribs were previously identified as being amenable to healing with cage rest and analgesics. Incomplete or greenstick fractures of most bones heal satisfactorily if the animal's activity is limited to a cage. Minimally displaced complete fractures of bones in paired bone systems, such as a diaphyseal fracture of the ulna when the radius is intact, do not require repair in many cases. Fractures of the vertebrae or skull without accompanying neurologic deficits likely do not benefit from repair versus cage confinement.

For fractures that require repair, there are a constantly expanding number of orthopedic devices that may be applied (Table 2), along with a seemingly infinite number of variations or configurations of some of those devices (eg, rigid versus circular skeletal fixators). For each given fracture configuration,

Table 2
Fixation devices for fractures

Devices/Techniques	Uses
External coaptation	Closed fractures distal to the elbow or stifle
IM pin (single)	Never
IM pin with full cerclage	Long oblique or spiral fractures
IM pin with external fixator	Many diaphyseal and metaphyseal fractures
Rush pin technique	Metaphyseal, physeal, and epiphyseal fractures
Tension band fixation	Avulsion or iatrogenic fractures of bony prominences
Interlocking IM nail	Most diaphyseal fracture configurations
External fixators	Most diaphyseal and metaphyseal fractures
Circular fixators	Most fractures (experience needed)
Bone plate (anatomic)	Most fracture configurations because of varied plate design
Bone plate and, rod	Buttressed fracture repairs
Ancillary devices	
Full cerclage wires	
Hemicerclage wires	
K-wires/crossed K-wires	
Lag screws	

Abbreviation: IM, intramedullary.

every available device should be considered in terms of its ability to control all the forces (bending, compression, shear, tension, and torsion) acting on the fracture; additionally, the overall strength [7] and ability of each fixation device to provide early rigid stability and anatomic reduction of joint surfaces and to allow early return to function should be considered. Experience and training provide mental snapshots (patterns) based on observation of similar fractures that have healed successfully (or not healed), providing the basis for a surgeon's choice from among the many devices available. If any particular fixation device does not provide resistance to any given force or does not provide sufficient overall strength to allow weight bearing during healing, the fixation choice is eliminated from consideration. Thus, the availability of the needed equipment and expertise is identified before attempting surgery, or referral is chosen if such equipment or expertise is not available. During surgery, if the primary choice for fixation cannot be applied (because of unanticipated difficulties during surgery), alternative acceptable fixation choices are already identified.

There are a number of devices listed as "ancillary" in Table 2 that may provide secondary support to "primary" devices but should never be the sole means of fixation of any fracture. Likewise, several devices commonly used in the past are no longer considered as acceptable methods of repair because of the high rates of complications associated with their use or better modern alternatives. The Schroeder-Thomas splint is still commonly used in general veterinary practice but is the most complication-prone and outdated device currently available. The extended use of the Schroeder-Thomas splint for fixation too often results in unacceptable joint contracture, osteoporosis, and muscle atrophy. Additionally, it is often inappropriately used to stabilize femoral and humeral fractures, resulting in increased rather than decreased motion at the fracture site. Multiple (stacked) intramedullary pin use has been advocated in the past for control of rotation in transverse fractures, but rotational resistance with this fixation technique is inadequate compared with most external skeletal fixation configurations or bone plates.

Regardless of the repair method chosen, the surgeon should plan and be familiar with the surgical approach. The surgeon should think through the entire procedure from start to finish before surgery as an aid in streamlining the repair procedure and anticipating repair needs. One frequent intraoperative decision faced occurs when the plan or fixation device identified before surgery cannot be used in the operating theater. This decision is often necessitated because of greater than expected comminution, unrecognized fissures, difficult fragment reduction, or life-threatening patient emergencies. Preoperative determination of acceptable fixation alternatives and availability of the equipment and expertise for those alternatives, as discussed previously, aids in switching fixation choices with a minimum of delay and difficulty.

BONE GRAFTS

Bone grafts provide a number of potential benefits to fracture healing and should be incorporated into the fracture repair if any question of the need for their properties exists [8]. They are useful to place in any gap in the fracture reduction during anatomic fragment reduction as well as to promote healing during arthrodesis of any joint or in the treatment of osteomyelitis or nonunion. Depending on the type and source of the graft, grafts may provide live osteoblasts, osteoinductive properties, osteoconductive properties, or mechanical support. Osteoinduction refers to the induction by protein mediators of living cells within the graft and osteoprogenitor cells within the recipient site to produce bone. These mediators are released from bone during resorption by osteoclasts and are known collectively as bone morphogenetic proteins (BMPs). Osteoconduction refers to the graft acting as a scaffold for recipient capillaries and cells to facilitate bone remodeling by osteoclast resorption and creation of new vascular channels, a process known as creeping substitution.

If the possible need for cancellous or cortical grafts has been identified during the preoperative planning stage, provisions for procuring these grafts before or during surgery should be made. Bone grafts commonly used in veterinary practice include cancellous autografts, corticocancellous autografts, and cortical allografts, although the use of commercial bone graft substitutes and cytokines seems to be increasing.

Cancellous and corticocancellous autografts are harvested from different sites (other than the fractured bone) in the same patient, and both provide cellular elements as well as osteoconductive and osteoinductive properties. There is obviously no antigenic stimulation by these autografts, and incorporation is generally quick. Cancellous bone grafts in the dog and cat can be harvested from any sizable metaphyseal area of a long bone. Corticocancellous grafts in the dog or cat are primarily harvested as whole ribs or iliac crest grafts that are then morselized to provide greater surface area and easier nutrient diffusion from the recipient site. Harvest should be accomplished in an aseptic fashion using separate instruments and preferably be performed by a separate surgical team other than that repairing the fracture. Cancellous and cortico-cancellous grafts may both be placed into infected sites, where they may die before contributing to the fracture repair but do not complicate the repair by sequestering.

Cortical bone grafts in the dog and cat are generally allografts harvested from donor animals being euthanized for other noninfectious reasons. Cortical allografts can be collected and stored in a sterile fashion or can be harvested without regard to sterile technique and then sterilized, preferably by ethylene oxide sterilization, and stored in a cooler or at room temperature. In either instance, removal of soft tissue and remaining marrow is important to limit the antigenic reaction to the graft. Cortical grafts do not provide living cellular elements but still retain osteoinductive and osteoconductive properties and can serve as mechanical support in large bone defects.

Complications after collection of autogenous cancellous graft are rare. Infection of the donor site, seroma formation, or fracture of the donor bone is a potential risk but is uncommon. Pneumothorax results if the pleural space is opened during collection of a rib for corticocancellous grafts but occurs less than 5% of the time in the author's experience.

There are an increasing number of synthetic bone graft materials on the market, which are composed of denatured animal bone (xenografts for the dog or cat); coral (hydroxyapatite); or, recently, bioactive ceramic containing calcium, sodium, silica, and phosphorus. Human recombinant BMP is also commercially available, if somewhat expensive, and has been used in the dog. These synthetic materials are advantageous in that they require no second harvest site and less subsequent preparation and surgical time; they can be placed in volume to fill large defects but are generally less potent than autogenous cancellous bone.

POSTOPERATIVE DECISIONS AND MANAGEMENT

Radiographs are taken immediately after surgery to allow assessment of the repair and serve for comparison with follow-up radiographs. Repairs should be critically reviewed by the surgeon to assess technical aspects of the repair and evaluate the chances for healing. Each repair should be evaluated in light of its ability to control the forces placed on the fracture: bending, compression, shear, tension, and torsion. Deficiencies in control of any of these forces should be dealt with immediately, preferably with the animal still under the anesthesia, rather than hoping against probable failure of the fixation.

After repair, the activity of all animals should be restricted to a cage or small run with good solid flooring when not directly observed by the client. Animals may be allowed brief activity outside when necessary and under controlled supervision. Veterinarians should be specific with simple and clear instructions about exercise restriction and patient care. Controlled physical therapy, including passive range of motion, is beneficial to maintain early joint range of motion and promote early limb use. Lately, underwater treadmills have begun to proliferate across referral centers and may prove useful for rehabilitation of the fracture patient. External coaptation or external fixators should be protected from damage by the patient, moisture, or other factors. Elizabethan collars may be necessary to prevent coaptation damage when the animal is not directly observed. Analgesia should be maintained in the postoperative period as previously discussed.

Radiographs of the fracture and repair are taken at frequent intervals to assess healing of the fracture. Fixation appliances should not be removed until complete healing is documented on radiographs, although staged disassembly of external fixators may be useful after a complete callus forms to facilitate remodeling. Early signs of healing include a periosteal reaction near the fracture, callus formation at the fracture site, minor resorption and remodeling of fragment ends, incorporation of fragments or bone graft, or primary bridging of a rigidly stable fracture with woven bone. Signs of complete healing on radiographs include bridging of bone or callus across fracture lines, disappearance of fracture lines, and callus resorption or remodeling after fracture bridging. Initial recheck radiographs are taken 4 weeks after surgery in young animals and 8 weeks after surgery in adult animals. Additional radiographic rechecks are taken at 4- or 8-week intervals to follow healing. It is not necessary to remove most modern orthopedic implants after healing, with the exception of external fixators.

PROBLEM FRACTURES

There are a number of fractures that may prove particularly difficult to manage for the inexperienced and experienced orthopedic surgeon alike. Distal radial fractures in small-breed dogs have a high incidence of nonunion and should be given rigid plate or external fixator stability at the outset, along with a possible (and recommended) cancellous autograft. These fractures should never be splinted or casted as the primary means of fixation under any circumstances. Salter fractures of the distal ulnar physis of immature dogs are difficult to see on initial radiographs but often result in premature closure and carpal valgus. The client should be warned of the possible development of such deformities any time an animal presents with distal forelimb trauma. Distal femoral fractures in immature dogs are prone to develop a condition known as "quadriceps tiedown" in which the stifle range of motion is lost and the animal often becomes non–weight-bearing lame on the limb as growth continues. Correction of the condition after its occurrence is difficult or impossible, and prevention by early return to function and diligent physical therapy is the best method of prevention. Open fractures must be carefully cleansed, cultured, and monitored for signs of osteomyelitis during healing because of the increased incidence of infection with these fractures. Nonunion or malunion fractures require expert knowledge of rigid fixation methods, bone deformity correction, and bone grafting to result in an adequate second attempt at healing. Finally, humeral fractures in dogs are generally more difficult to correct than other long bones because of the shape of the bone, deep muscle coverage of the bone, and proximity to the body. Such options as a medial approach for plating and use of hybrid skeletal fixators can prove beneficial for treatment of these fractures but require extensive experience.

References

[1] Selcer BA, Buttrick M, Barstad R, et al. The incidence of thoracic trauma in dogs with skeletal injury. J Small Anim Pract 1987;28:21–7.

[2] Olsen D, Renberg W, Hauptman JG, et al. Clinical management of flail chest in dogs and cats: a retrospective study of 24 cases (1989–1999). J Am Anim Hosp Assoc 2002;38: 315–20.

[3] Selcer BA. Urinary tract trauma associated with pelvic trauma. J Am Anim Hosp Assoc 1982;18:785–93.

[4] Reiss AJ, McKiernan BC, Wingfield WE. Myocardial injury secondary to blunt thoracic trauma in dogs: diagnosis and treatment. Compend Contin Educ Pract Vet 2002;24: 944–51.

[5] Aron DN, Palmer RH, Johnson AL. Biologic strategies and a balanced concept for repair of highly comminuted long bone fractures. Compend Contin Educ Pract Vet 1995;17:35–49.

[6] Rochat MC, Payne JT. Your options in managing long-bone fractures in dogs and cats. Veterinary Medicine 1993;88:946–56.

[7] Muir P, Johnson KA, Markel MD. Area moment of inertia for comparison of implant cross-sectional geometry and bending stiffness. Vet Comp Orthop Traumatol 1995;8:146–52.

[8] Fitch R, Kerwin S, Sinibaldi KR, et al. Bone autografts and allograft in dogs. Compend Contin Educ Pract Vet 1997;19:558–75.

Vet Clin Small Anim 35 (2005) 1155–1167

ELSEVIER
SAUNDERS

VETERINARY CLINICS
SMALL ANIMAL PRACTICE

Common Malignant Musculoskeletal Neoplasms of Dogs and Cats

Ruthanne Chun, DVM

University of Wisconsin-Madison School of Veterinary Medicine, 2015 Linden Drive, Madison, WI 53706, USA

TUMORS OF THE LONG BONES OF THE APPENDICULAR SKELETON

Appendicular osteosarcoma in dogs

Because a thorough review of canine osteosarcoma (OSA), the most common primary bone tumor in dogs, recently was published, only the clinical highlights of canine OSA are included in this article [1]. Appendicular skeletal OSA is typically seen in young or middle-aged to older, large to giant breeds, with male species being overrepresented in most reports [2–7].

Clinical signs, history, and physical examination findings of a distal radial, proximal humeral, distal femoral, or proximal tibial lesion are usually highly suspicious for OSA; a definitive diagnosis is obtained through histopathologic evaluation of a core or surgical biopsy. Fine-needle aspiration may help differentiate OSA from an inflammatory or metastatic lesion. Other recommended diagnostic tests include a complete blood count (CBC), chemistry profile, urinalysis, three-view thoracic radiographs (metastasis check), and radiographs of the primary lesion. Nuclear scintigraphy is a sensitive imaging modality that may identify early bony metastases [8–11]. Prognostic factors reported to affect survival adversely include any elevation in alkaline phosphatase at the time of diagnosis, tumor location on the proximal humerus or scapula, young or old age at diagnosis (dogs between 7 and 10 years had the longest survival times), the presence of metastatic disease, histologic subtype, histologic grade 3, and large tumor volume or area [3,5,7,10,12–16]. OSA that involves the bones distal to the antebrachiocarpal and tarsocrural joints may have a less aggressive biologic behavior, but the treatment recommendations for OSA at these sites remain as described later [17].

The biologic behavior of appendicular OSA is aggressive, with most dogs dying of metastases within months of diagnosis. The standard of care involves surgery to remove the painful tumor followed by chemotherapy in an attempt

E-mail address: chunr@svm.vetmed.wisc.edu

0195-5616/05/$ – see front matter
doi:10.1016/j.cvsm.2005.05.004

to address metastatic disease. Cisplatin and carboplatin are reportedly equally effective against metastases; four to six doses typically are recommended [3,18–22]. The longest reported median survival time with surgery and platinum-based chemotherapy was 413 days [20]. One study that used surgery and five doses of doxorubicin administered every other week reported a median survival of 366 days [4]. Although the longest reported median survival of 540 days was observed with surgery plus doxorubicin and cisplatin combination chemotherapy, other studies using the same combination have failed to demonstrate similarly prolonged survival [6,23]. Unfortunately, chemotherapy is ineffective in the face of gross disease [24].

Less traditional therapies that involve limb sparing through surgery or radiation therapy have been well described [25–29]. Sites most amenable to limb-sparing surgeries include the distal radius and the proximal scapula [26,27,30,31]. Distal radial lesions may be resected and allografted without inhibiting limb functionality. Likewise, removal of the proximal half of the scapula is associated with good to excellent limb function. Administration of high doses of radiation one time, either in conjunction with surgery or alone, is another option that may become more widely available in the future [28,29]. Because limb-sparing options do not address metastatic disease, chemotherapy after surgery is still recommended as standard of care.

Palliative therapies (ie, therapies that improve quality of life but do not attempt to treat the metastatic disease) include medical pain management, amputation alone, or radiation therapy. Commonly recommended drugs include nonsteroidal anti-inflammatory drugs (eg, carprofen, etogesic, or piroxicam) alone or in combination with acetaminophen or acetaminophen with codeine. A fentanyl patch may be indicated for animals with severe pain whose owners decline euthanasia. Bisphosphonates also have been reported to provide palliation in dogs with OSA [32]. Although little information exists in peer-reviewed literature regarding the dose and efficacy of the many bisphosphonates available for clinical use, many veterinary studies have been undertaken and are awaiting publication [33]. Because these drugs have been shown to inhibit the growth of canine OSA cell lines and because they are widely used in human medicine to control bone pain, bisphosphonates hold potential to be effective in the definitive and palliative management of OSA [33,34]. Issues that remain to be clarified include which bisphosphonate to use, route of administration, and dosage. A recent publication offered further depth on bisphosphonates [33]. Radiation therapy delivered in three or four large fractions improved limb function and quality of life in 75% of patients, with duration of relief typically ranging from 2 to 4 months [35–37]. Amputation of the affected limb can provide significant relief from the painful bony tumor and may prolong survival. Survival after palliative therapy tends to be short, however, with reported median of 4 to 6 months [2,5,21,35,37]. Dogs treated palliatively with radiation or medical management are usually euthanized because of recurrence of pain at the tumor site; dogs treated with amputation alone are euthanized because of rapid development of metastases.

Osteosarcoma in cats

OSA is the most common primary bone tumor in cats and accounts for more than 70% of all reported primary bone tumors in cats [38,39]. Middle-aged to older cats are most frequently reported, although cats as young as 3.5 months have been reported [39]. Appendicular and axial OSAs seem to be equally distributed, although one study cited 68% of the cases arising on the appendicular skeleton [38–40]. Within the appendicular skeleton, the rear legs are more commonly affected than the forelegs. Regardless of primary site, the biologic behavior of feline OSA is locally invasive but slow to metastasize [38–40]. Even so, staging with radiographs of the primary lesion and thorax is advised to rule out metastasis, and a presurgical evaluation with a CBC, chemistry profile, and urinalysis is warranted to rule out concurrent disease. Aggressive surgical resection (ie, amputation) is often curative. If complete resection is impossible (eg, because of axial skeletal involvement), radiation therapy is a reasonable option, although no studies document the value of this treatment. Few reports are available on the use of chemotherapy for cats with unresectable OSA. Combination therapy of vincristine, cyclophosphamide, and methotrexate was associated with partial remission in a cat with pelvic OSA. Carboplatin was used in two cats with extraskeletal OSA, one of which experienced a decrease in tumor size during therapy, which allowed for a curative surgery [40–42].

Fibrosarcoma

Although fibrosarcoma (FSA) is a relatively common extraskeletal malignancy, it is a relatively uncommon primary bone tumor in dogs [43–47]. Appendicular FSA is an important differential for appendicular OSA, because the presenting complaints, physical examination findings, and radiographic findings are similar to those with OSA. Because cytologic analysis of a fine-needle aspirate may not differentiate between FSA and OSA, a biopsy is warranted. An important aspect of histopathologic assessment of soft tissue origin FSA is tumor grade [48]. Grade 1 or 2 FSA is unlikely to metastasize; long-term control or cure is likely with aggressive surgery with or without radiation therapy [43,46,49–51]. A grade 3, or high-grade, FSA is more likely to metastasize, and chemotherapy is warranted as adjuvant therapy [51]. Whether this grading system is valid for bone origin FSA remains to be determined. The inability to reduce the tumor to microscopic disease surgically, especially at the time of the first therapeutic surgical attempt, is a poor prognostic factor regardless of grade [51,52]. In the event of an unresectable FSA, radiation therapy or chemotherapy is indicated. For microscopic local residual disease, radiation therapy is a highly effective treatment option [45]. Animals with metastatic FSA should be treated with chemotherapy. Unfortunately, few data are available regarding what chemotherapy protocol is most effective against metastatic FSA.

Primary FSA of the bone is rare in cats. A more common scenario in this species is FSA, or other soft tissue sarcoma, that arises at the site of a vaccination. This tumor type is discussed later in this article.

Chondrosarcoma

Chondrosarcoma (CSA) accounts for approximately 10% of all primary bone tumors in dogs [53]. Large-breed dogs are most commonly affected [53]. CSA is another important differential for a dog with a primary bone tumor; a biopsy often provides a definitive diagnosis. The three most common sites of CSA in the skeleton are rib, appendicular skeleton, and nasal cavity [53]. The biologic behavior of CSA seems to be locally invasive and slow to metastasize [43,53,54]. Aggressive surgical resection is the treatment of choice with the goal of long-term survival or cure [43,53,54]. Dogs with appendicular CSA should have an amputation performed; CSA at other skeletal sites should be similarly aggressively resected. Information regarding adjuvant radiation therapy or chemotherapy for incompletely resected or metastatic CSA is lacking.

Primary bone CSA is a rare tumor in cats. Because local disease is the most life-threatening aspect of these tumors in cats, aggressive surgical resection is the primary treatment recommendation.

TUMORS OF THE AXIAL SKELETON

Axial osteosarcoma in dogs

As with appendicular disease, axial OSA tends to affect large-breed dogs. Middle-aged to older dogs are usually affected. The mandible and maxilla are the most common sites, although any portion of the axial skeleton can be involved [55]. The biologic behavior of axial OSA is as aggressive as appendicular OSA, with the notable exception of mandibular OSA. Mandibular OSA does not seem to be as rapidly metastatic; 71% of the dogs in one study treated with mandibulectomy alone were still alive and free from their disease 1 year after treatment with surgery alone [56]. The current standard of care involves surgical resection of the affected site followed by chemotherapy with four to six doses of a platinum (cisplatin or carboplatin) protocol. Doxorubicin as a single agent has not been evaluated for the treatment of canine axial OSA.

As with appendicular OSA, palliative therapy for axial OSA involves medical pain management or radiation therapy. If necessary, medical pain management is recommended as in a previous section. The use of radiation therapy also has been reported for dogs with axial OSA. Although it seems that definitive therapy may be associated with longer survival times than palliative therapy, more studies are necessary to elucidate specifics [55,57]. Most dogs with axial OSA are euthanized because of complications associated with the primary tumor [14,43,46,54–63]. Median survival times for dogs with axial OSA tend to be shorter than for appendicular OSA because of the difficulty in completely resecting the primary tumor.

Multilobular tumor of bone (multilobular osteochondrosarcoma)

Multilobular tumor of bone has a characteristic radiographic appearance that allows for a strong suspicion of this tumor based on minimally invasive diagnostics [64,65]. Histologically, the tumor is a multilobular mass; the lobules are demarcated by fibrovascular stroma and have a central area of cartilage or bone that may be calcified or ossified [66]. The lengthy name is based on the gross and microscopic lobular appearance with production of cartilage or bone in the central areas. Multilobular tumor of bone usually arises from the flat bones of the skull and is most often reported in middle-aged to older dogs, although there are rare reports of this tumor in cats [64,66–69].

Most animals with multilobular tumor of bone present for evaluation of a slowly progressive, firm mass on the skull. Radiographically, the tumor has well-defined borders, a coarsely granular appearance, and stippled to nodular mineralized opacities [65]. The characteristic "popcorn ball" appearance supports a clinical diagnosis of multilobular tumor of bone [64,66]. Because CT imaging offers superior bone detail, cross-sectional imaging may be helpful before recommending and planning therapy.

Multilobular tumor of bone is locally invasive, and ≤60% metastasize to the lungs, although only 10% of cases have metastases at the time of diagnosis. The median time to metastasis is 420 to 542 days [64,66]. The most important prognostic factor is tumor location; tumors located on the mandible were more easily excisable, and median survival time in dogs affected at this site was 1487 days [66]. Other prognostic factors are histologic grade and whether the tumor was completely excised [66]. Tumor grade is based on subjective and objective data. The reader is referred elsewhere for a complete description of the grading scheme [66].

Surgery is the treatment of choice for multilobular tumor of bone. Aggressive resection of the affected site is typically well tolerated and the best chance for cure [64,66,69,70]. After surgery, median survival times range from 630 to 797 days [64,66]. Unfortunately, there is little information in the literature to guide clinicians in treatment decisions beyond surgical excision. Metastatic disease warrants chemotherapy; however, the onset of metastases is typically late in the course of disease. Animals with incompletely resected tumors are more likely to experience recurrent disease and die because of local complications. Radiation therapy is likely to prolong the disease-free interval.

Rib, vertebral, and pelvic tumors

Primary bone tumors that involve the rib, vertebral body, and pelvis are rare in dogs and cats. The most common primary rib tumors are OSA, FSA, and CSA [43,54]. The most common primary vertebral tumors are OSA and FSA [46]. The most common primary pelvic tumor is OSA [49]. The reader is directed to the previous sections for discussion on management of specific tumor types.

Plasma cell tumors

Although plasma cell tumors are rare and multiple myeloma is more often considered a systemic disease rather than a primary bone tumor, they are important differentials when a bone tumor is suspected.

Multiple myeloma

Multiple myeloma is considered a systemic plasma cell malignancy that arises within the bone marrow. This tumor is covered in this article because osteolytic bone lesions are a hallmark. The disease is rare in cats and is uncommon in dogs. It accounts for 8% of all canine hematopoietic tumors and affects older dogs, with no breed or sex predilection.

Often animals present for care because of clinical signs associated with excessive immunoglobulin production by the malignant cells. The immunoglobulin (Ig), typically IgG or IgA, can cause multiple problems for the animal. Infection is a major issue because excessive production of the tumor Ig inhibits production of normal Ig; patients are considered to be immunologic cripples. Hyperviscosity syndrome arises secondary to the massive amounts of paraprotein present. Heart failure, neurologic abnormalities, kidney failure, and retinopathies are all possible sequelae of hyperviscosity. Hemorrhagic diatheses are common. Animals may present with nonspecific signs of weakness, polyuria and polydipsia, lethargy, or lack of appetite. More specific signs include pain, bleeding, seizures, or mental dullness or signs caused by a compressive lesion or fracture.

Because the presenting complaint is often nonspecific, a CBC, chemistry profile, and urinalysis are typically obtained first. The CBC may reveal anemia, thrombocytopenia, or leukopenia. The chemistry profile is usually helpful; ≥90% of patients show hyperglobulinemia, 16% have hypercalcemia, and 33% of patients have evidence of azotemia [71]. Serum electrophoresis should be performed to characterize the hyperglobulinemia; most animals with myeloma have a monoclonal gammopathy [71]. Although up to 40% of patients have Bence-Jones proteins within the urine (light-chains of myeloma proteins), routine urinalysis does not always detect this abnormality [71]. The best method for detection of Bence-Jones proteinuria is heat precipitation and electrophoresis [71]. Other tests recommended in the diagnosis and staging of multiple myeloma include bone marrow aspirate, survey skeletal radiographs, and biopsy or fine-needle aspirate of the characteristic osteolytic bone lesions. Diagnosis of multiple myeloma is based on finding two or more of the following factors: (1) bone marrow plasmacytosis, (2) presence of osteolytic bone lesions, (3) monoclonal gammopathy, and (4) Bence-Jones proteinuria [71]. Hypercalcemia, Bence-Jones proteinuria, and extensive osteolytic bone lesions are all negative prognostic factors [71,72].

Multiple myeloma is a gratifying tumor to treat in dogs because it responds quickly and the patient's life is significantly longer and of better quality than without chemotherapy. It is important to remember that cures are rare and the disease ultimately relapses. A combination chemotherapy protocol of melphalan and prednisone is recommended. Median survival time in dogs treated for multiple myeloma is 540 days [71]. Few treated cases of feline multiple myeloma have been reported, but median survivals are typically shorter at 2 to 3 months; however, some cats survive more than 1 year with the disease [73,74].

Solitary osseous plasmacytoma

Solitary osseous plasmacytomas (SOPs) are plasma cell tumors that involve a single osseous site. Large, middle-aged to older dogs are usually affected, although cases in animals as young as 1 year of age have been reported [75]. Unlike multiple myeloma, which typically causes multiple bony lesions, SOPs do not produce immunoglobulin, and the myriad problems associated with hyperviscosity syndrome are not seen with SOP.

Animals with SOP present with signs of bone pain or sequelae to a bony lesion (eg, lameness or neurologic deficits secondary to a vertebral lesion) [75]. Radiographs of the painful site typically show bony lysis with little to no new bone proliferation [75]. Fine-needle aspirate or biopsy of the lytic area is usually diagnostic for plasma cell tumor [75]; all patients with suspected SOP should be evaluated thoroughly with a CBC, chemistry profile, urinalysis, and survey radiographs of the thoracic and lumbar spine in an attempt to rule out multiple myeloma.

Because this tumor is localized, surgical resection and radiation therapy are excellent treatment options. An unknown percentage of dogs with SOP develop multiple myeloma, and the role of chemotherapy in the management of SOP remains unclear. In four dogs treated with chemotherapy and radiation therapy, the survival times ranged from 4 to 65 months [75].

Metastatic bone tumors

Metastatic bone tumors are rare but important differentials in animals with bone tumors. The most common carcinomas to metastasize to bone are tumors that arise in the mammary gland, bladder (ie, transitional cell carcinoma), and prostate [47,50]. OSA also has been reported to metastasize to bone, but in this setting the metastatic lesions are not likely to be the cause for the initial presentation [8,10,76]. As with primary bone tumors, the radiographic appearance of metastatic bone tumors involves bony lysis and new bone proliferation. Metastatic bone tumors are more likely to involve the diaphysis than are primary bone tumors. To exclude the possibility of a metastatic bone tumor, a thorough physical examination, including rectal examination, is warranted in any animal that presents with a bone tumor.

Treatment of metastatic bone tumors is rarely rewarding. Surgery is often not a realistic option because of the systemic extent of disease, and chemotherapy is unlikely to significantly impact the disease. Radiation therapy may be used palliatively to diminish pain and prolong survival [50,77,78].

TUMORS OF THE JOINTS

Synovial cell sarcoma

Synovial cell sarcoma is typically believed to be the most common primary joint tumor in dogs, and it is a rare tumor in cats [79–82]. While the age, sex, and breed affected biologic behavior and treatment recommendations are unknown in cats, one case report suggested that cats may be effectively treated with aggressive surgery alone [80]. The remainder of this discussion focuses on dogs.

The median age at diagnosis is 9 years, although reported ages range from 3 to 15 years [79,81,82]. The tumor can arise within any joint, although the stifle is the most common site [79]. The biologic behavior is locally invasive; metastases to lymph nodes, lungs, spleen, or brain are evident in approximately 8% to 22% of cases at diagnosis, and ultimately 41% go on to other sites [79,81].

A diagnosis of synovial cell sarcoma is suspected based on radiographic evidence of bony lysis plus or minus periosteal new bone formation and involvement of >1 articular bone surface [79]. Up to 54% of cases for which radiographs are obtained show no bony changes [81]. Fine-needle aspiration may offer a preliminary diagnosis, but surgical biopsy is recommended for definitive diagnosis. The value of prognostic information based on tumor grade, cytokeratin staining, and histologic classification is questionable [79,81]. A more significant prognostic factor is whether the lesion can be completely excised surgically [81]. Before definitive surgery, staging of dogs with synovial cell sarcoma should include a thoracic metastasis check, fine-needle aspirates of the regional lymph nodes, and overall patient health assessment with a CBC, chemistry profile, and urinalysis. With complete resection and no evidence of metastasis before surgery, median survival is more than 2 years.

Other joint tumors

Malignancies of the joint other than synovial cell sarcoma are rare. Other primary tumors, such as OSA, lymphoma, histiocytic sarcoma, synovial myxoma, malignant fibrous histiocytoma, FSA, CSA, and undifferentiated sarcoma, have been reported [82–84]. The joints are infrequent sites of metastasis [85]. Because of the paucity of literature regarding the clinical management of animals with joint tumors other than synovial cell sarcoma, the reader is directed toward discussions of the tumors that arise from more typical sites for guidance on treatment options.

SOFT TISSUE TUMORS OF THE MUSCULOSKELETAL SYSTEM

Injection site sarcomas

Vaccine site sarcomas of cats recently have been reviewed thoroughly [86,87]. Briefly, vaccine site sarcomas are highly locally invasive and metastasize in up to 23% of patients [88]. Aggressive surgical resection is the mainstay of therapy; however, chemotherapy and radiation therapy prolong survival times and are important components of patient management [88–95]. Even with this aggressive therapy, cures are rare. Suspected vaccine site sarcomas recently were described in dogs [96]. There are no reports on the biologic behavior of these tumors in dogs. Whether injection site sarcomas in dogs will become a more widely recognized phenomenon remains to be seen.

Hemangiosarcoma

Hemangiosarcoma may arise as primary bone tumor in dogs or cats, but a more common scenario that involves the musculoskeletal system is primary muscular disease [39,62,97–101]. The biologic behavior of hemangiosarcoma that involves the musculoskeletal system is locally invasive and highly metastatic [101]. Diagnostic evaluation should include not only diagnostic imaging and biopsy of the primary lesion but also thoracic and abdominal radiographs and abdominal ultrasound to stage the disease. A CBC, chemistry profile, and urinalysis should be obtained to evaluate the overall health of the patient. Animals with evidence of metastasis on staging evaluation have a poorer prognosis, because patients who have measurable disease after surgery have a significantly shorter survival period than patients who have no detectable disease postoperatively [102,103]. Adjuvant chemotherapy with a doxorubicin-based protocol is recommended. Because the literature is scant regarding surgical resection of musculoskeletal hemangiosarcoma followed by chemotherapy, it is difficult to provide accurate survival data. Extrapolation from reports of treating splenic hemangiosarcoma with surgery followed by chemotherapy suggests that patients rendered down to microscopic disease have median survival times of 7 to 8 months [102,103]. Patients with macroscopic disease after surgery have median survival times of 2 to 3 months [102,103].

References

[1] Chun R, de Lorimier LP. Update on the biology and management of canine osteosarcoma. Vet Clin North Am Small Anim Pract 2003;33:491–516[vi.].

[2] Thompson JP, Fugent MJ. Evaluation of survival times after limb amputation, with and without subsequent administration of cisplatin, for treatment of appendicular osteosarcoma in dogs: 30 cases (1979–1990). J Am Vet Med Assoc 1992;200:531–3.

[3] Bergman PJ, MacEwen EG, Kurzman ID, et al. Amputation and carboplatin for treatment of dogs with osteosarcoma: 48 cases (1991 to 1993). J Vet Intern Med 1996;10:76–81.

[4] Berg J, Weinstein MJ, Springfield DS, et al. Results of surgery and doxorubicin chemotherapy in dogs with osteosarcoma. J Am Vet Med Assoc 1995;206:1555–60.

[5] Spodnick GJ, Berg J, Rand WM, et al. Prognosis for dogs with appendicular osteosarcoma treated by amputation alone: 162 cases (1978–1988). J Am Vet Med Assoc 1992;200:995–9.

[6] Berg J, Gebhardt MC, Rand WM. Effect of timing of postoperative chemotherapy on survival of dogs with osteosarcoma. Cancer 1997;79:1343–50.

[7] Misdorp W, Hart AA. Some prognostic and epidemiologic factors in canine osteosarcoma. J Natl Cancer Inst 1979;62:537–45.

[8] Forrest LJ, Thrall DE. Bone scintigraphy for metastasis detection in canine osteosarcoma. Vet Radiol Ultrasound 1994;35:124–30.

[9] Jaffe N, Pearson P, Yasko AW, et al. Single and multiple metachronous osteosarcoma tumors after therapy. Cancer 2003;98:2457–66.

[10] Forrest LJ, Dodge RK, Page RL, et al. Relationship between quantitative tumor scintigraphy and time to metastasis in dogs with osteosarcoma. J Nucl Med 1992;33:1542–7.

[11] Wolff RK, Merickel BS, Rebar AH, et al. Comparison of bone scans and radiography for detecting bone neoplasms in dogs exposed to 238PuO2. Am J Vet Res 1980;41:1804–7.

[12] Ehrhart N, Dernell WS, Hoffmann WE, et al. Prognostic importance of alkaline phosphatase activity in serum from dogs with appendicular osteosarcoma: 75 cases (1990–1996). J Am Vet Med Assoc 1998;213:1002–6.

[13] Garzotto CK, Berg J, Hoffmann WE, et al. Prognostic significance of serum alkaline phosphatase activity in canine appendicular osteosarcoma. J Vet Intern Med 2000;14:587–92.

[14] Hammer AS, Weeren FR, Weisbrode SE, et al. Prognostic factors in dogs with osteosarcomas of the flat or irregular bones. J Am Anim Hosp Assoc 1995;31:321–6.

[15] Kirpensteijn J, Kik M, Rutteman G, et al. Prognostic significance of a new histologic grading system for canine osteosarcoma. Vet Pathol 2002;39:240–6.
[16] Brodey RS, Abt DA. Results of surgical treatment in 65 dogs with osteosarcoma. J Am Vet Med Assoc 1976;168:1032–5.
[17] Gamblin RM, Straw RC, Powers BE, et al. Primary osteosarcoma distal to the antebrachiocarpal and tarsocrural joints in nine dogs (1980–1992). J Am Anim Hosp Assoc 1995;31:86–90.
[18] Shapiro W, Fossum TW, Kitchell BE, et al. Use of cisplatin for treatment of appendicular osteosarcoma in dogs. J Am Vet Med Assoc 1988;192:507–11.
[19] Berg J, Weinstein MJ, Schelling SH, et al. Treatment of dogs with osteosarcoma by administration of cisplatin after amputation or limb-sparing surgery: 22 cases (1987–1990). J Am Vet Med Assoc 1992;200:2005–8.
[20] Kraegel SA, Madewell BR, Simonson E, et al. Osteogenic sarcoma and cisplatin chemotherapy in dogs: 16 cases (1986–1989). J Am Vet Med Assoc 1991;199:1057–9.
[21] Mauldin GN, Matus RE, Withrow SJ, et al. Canine osteosarcoma: treatment by amputation versus amputation and adjuvant chemotherapy using doxorubicin and cisplatin. J Vet Intern Med 1988;2:177–80.
[22] Straw RC, Withrow SJ, Richter SL, et al. Amputation and cisplatin for treatment of canine osteosarcoma. J Vet Intern Med 1991;5:205–10.
[23] Chun R, Kurzman ID, Couto CG, et al. Cisplatin and doxorubicin combination chemotherapy for the treatment of canine osteosarcoma: a pilot study. J Vet Intern Med 2000;14:495–8.
[24] Ogilvie GK, Straw RC, Jameson VJ, et al. Evaluation of single-agent chemotherapy for treatment of clinically evident osteosarcoma metastases in dogs: 45 cases (1987–1991). J Am Vet Med Assoc 1993;202:304–6.
[25] Trout NJ, Pavletic MM, Kraus KH. Partial scapulectomy for management of sarcomas in three dogs and two cats. J Am Vet Med Assoc 1995;207:585–7.
[26] Rovesti GL, Bascucci M, Schmidt K, et al. Limb sparing using a double bone-transport technique for treatment of a distal tibial osteosarcoma in a dog. Vet Surg 2002;31:70–7.
[27] LaRue SM, Withrow SJ, Powers BE, et al. Limb-sparing treatment for osteosarcoma in dogs. J Am Vet Med Assoc 1989;195:1734–44.
[28] Liptak JM, Dernell WS, Lascelles BD, et al. Intraoperative extracorporeal irradiation for limb sparing in 13 dogs. Vet Surg 2004;33:446–56.
[29] Farese JP, Milner R, Thompson MS, et al. Stereotactic radiosurgery for treatment of osteosarcomas involving the distal portions of the limbs in dogs. J Am Vet Med Assoc 2004;225:1567–72, 1548.
[30] O'Brien M, Straw R, Withrow S. Recent advances in the treatment of canine appendicular osteosarcoma. Compendium on Continuing Education for the Practicing Veterinarian 1993;15:939–45.
[31] Morello E, Buracco P, Martano M, et al. Bone allografts and adjuvant cisplatin for the treatment of canine appendicular osteosarcoma in 18 dogs. J Small Anim Pract 2001;42:61–6.
[32] Tomlin JL, Sturgeon C, Pead MJ, et al. Use of the bisphosphonate drug alendronate for palliative management of osteosarcoma in two dogs. Vet Rec 2000;147:129–32.
[33] Milner RJ, Farese J, Henry CJ, et al. Bisphosphonates and cancer. J Vet Intern Med 2004;18:597–604.
[34] Poirier VJ, Huelsmeyer MK, Kurzman ID. The bisphosphonates alendronate and zoledronate are inhibitors of canine and human osteosarcoma cell growth in vitro. Veterinary and Comparative Oncology 2003;1:207–15.
[35] Green EM, Adams WM, Forrest LJ. Four fraction palliative radiotherapy for osteosarcoma in 24 dogs. J Am Anim Hosp Assoc 2002;38:445–51.
[36] Ramirez O III, Dodge RK, Page RL, et al. Palliative radiotherapy of appendicular osteosarcoma in 95 dogs. Vet Radiol Ultrasound 1999;40:517–22.

[37] McEntee MC, Page RL, Novotney CA, et al. Palliative radiotherapy for canine appendicular osteosarcoma. Vet Radiol Ultrasound 1993;34:367–70.

[38] Heldmann E, Anderson MA, Wagner-Mann C. Feline osteosarcoma: 145 cases (1990–1995). J Am Anim Hosp Assoc 2000;36:518–21.

[39] Quigley P, Leedale A. Tumors involving bone in the domestic cat: a review of fifty-eight cases. Vet Pathol 1983;20:670–86.

[40] Bitetto WV, Patnaik AK, Schrader SC, et al. Osteosarcoma in cats: 22 cases (1974–1984). J Am Vet Med Assoc 1987;190:91–3.

[41] Dhaliwal RS, Johnson TO, Kitchell BE. Primary extraskeletal hepatic osteosarcoma in a cat. J Am Vet Med Assoc 2003;222:340–2, 316.

[42] Spugnini EP, Ruslander D, Bartolazzi A. Extraskeletal osteosarcoma in a cat. J Am Vet Med Assoc 2001;219:60–2, 49.

[43] Pirkey-Ehrhart N, Withrow SJ, Straw RC, et al. Primary rib tumors in 54 dogs. J Am Anim Hosp Assoc 1995;31:65–9.

[44] Ciekot PA, Powers BE, Withrow SJ, et al. Histologically low-grade, yet biologically high-grade, fibrosarcomas of the mandible and maxilla in dogs: 25 cases (1982–1991). J Am Vet Med Assoc 1994;204:610–5.

[45] Forrest LJ, Chun R, Adams WM, et al. Postoperative radiotherapy for canine soft tissue sarcoma. J Vet Intern Med 2000;14:578–82.

[46] Dernell WS, Van Vechten BJ, Straw RC, et al. Outcome following treatment of vertebral tumors in 20 dogs (1986–1995). J Am Anim Hosp Assoc 2000;36:245–51.

[47] Cooley DM, Waters DJ. Skeletal neoplasms of small dogs: a retrospective study and literature review. J Am Anim Hosp Assoc 1997;33:11–23.

[48] Powers BE, Hoopes PJ, Ehrhart EJ. Tumor diagnosis, grading, and staging. Semin Vet Med Surg (Small Anim) 1995;10:158–67.

[49] Straw RC, Withrow SJ, Powers BE. Partial or total hemipelvectomy in the management of sarcomas in nine dogs and two cats. Vet Surg 1992;21:183–8.

[50] McEntee MC. Radiation therapy in the management of bone tumors. Vet Clin North Am Small Anim Pract 1997;27:131–8.

[51] Dernell WS, Withrow SJ, Kuntz CA, et al. Principles of treatment for soft tissue sarcoma. Clin Tech Small Anim Pract 1998;13:59–64.

[52] Kuntz CA, Dernell WS, Powers BE, et al. Prognostic factors for surgical treatment of soft-tissue sarcomas in dogs: 75 cases (1986–1996). J Am Vet Med Assoc 1997;211:1147–51.

[53] Popovitch CA, Weinstein MJ, Goldschmidt MH, et al. Chondrosarcoma: a retrospective study of 97 dogs (1987–1990). J Am Anim Hosp Assoc 1994;30:81–5.

[54] Matthiesen DT, Clark GN, Orsher RJ, et al. En bloc resection of primary rib tumors in 40 dogs. Vet Surg 1992;21:201–4.

[55] Heyman SJ, Diefenderfer DL, Goldschmidt MH, et al. Canine axial skeletal osteosarcoma: a retrospective study of 116 cases (1986–1989). Vet Surg 1992;21:304–10.

[56] Straw RC, Powers BE, Klausner J, et al. Canine mandibular osteosarcoma: 51 cases (1980–1992). J Am Anim Hosp Assoc 1996;32:257–62.

[57] Dickerson ME, Page RL, LaDue TA, et al. Retrospective analysis of axial skeleton osteosarcoma in 22 large-breed dogs. J Vet Intern Med 2001;15:120–4.

[58] Kosovsky JK, Matthiesen DT, Marretta SM, et al. Results of partial mandibulectomy for the treatment of oral tumors in 142 dogs. Vet Surg 1991;20:397–401.

[59] Schwarz P, Withrow S, Curtis C, et al. Mandibular resection as a treatment for oral cancer in 81 dogs. J Am Anim Hosp Assoc 1991;27:601–10.

[60] Schwarz P, Withrow S, Curtis C, et al. Partial maxillary resection as a treatment for oral cancer in 61 dogs. J Am Anim Hosp Assoc 1991;27:617–24.

[61] Wallace J, Matthiesen DT, Patnaik AK. Hemimaxillectomy for the treatment of oral tumors in 69 dogs. Vet Surg 1992;21:337–41.

[62] Feeney DA, Johnston GR, Grindem CB, et al. Malignant neoplasia of canine ribs: clinical, radiographic, and pathologic findings. J Am Vet Med Assoc 1982;180:927–33.

[63] Moore GE, Mathey WS, Eggers JS, et al. Osteosarcoma in adjacent lumbar vertebrae in a dog. J Am Vet Med Assoc 2000;217:1038–40, 1008.

[64] Straw RC, LeCouteur RA, Powers BE, et al. Multilobular osteochondrosarcoma of the canine skull: 16 cases (1978–1988). J Am Vet Med Assoc 1989;195:1764–9.

[65] Hathcock JT, Newton JC. Computed tomographic characteristics of multilobular tumor of bone involving the cranium in 7 dogs and zygomatic arch in 2 dogs. Vet Radiol Ultrasound 2000;41:214–7.

[66] Dernell WS, Straw RC, Cooper MF, et al. Multilobular osteochondrosarcoma in 39 dogs: 1979–1993. J Am Anim Hosp Assoc 1998;34:11–8.

[67] Morton D. Chondrosarcoma arising in a multilobular chondroma in a cat. J Am Vet Med Assoc 1985;186:804–6.

[68] Yildiz F, Gurel A, Yesildere T, et al. Frontal chondrosarcoma in a cat. J Vet Sci 2003;4: 193–4.

[69] O'Brien MG, Withrow SJ, Straw RC, et al. Total and partial orbitectomy for the treatment of periorbital tumors in 24 dogs and 6 cats: a retrospective study. Vet Surg 1996;25:471–9.

[70] Moissonnier P, Devauchelle P, Delisle F. Cranioplasty after en bloc resection of calvarial chondroma rodens in two dogs. J Small Anim Pract 1997;38:358–63.

[71] Matus RE, Leifer CE, MacEwen EG, et al. Prognostic factors for multiple myeloma in the dog. J Am Vet Med Assoc 1986;188:1288–92.

[72] Vail DM. Plasma cell neoplasms. In: Withrow SJ, MacEwen EG, editors. Small animal clinical oncology. 3rd edition. Philadelphia: WB Saunders; 2001. p. 626–38.

[73] Fan TM, Kitchell BE, Dhaliwal RS, et al. Hematological toxicity and therapeutic efficacy of lomustine in 20 tumor-bearing cats: critical assessment of a practical dosing regimen. J Am Anim Hosp Assoc 2002;38:357–63.

[74] Bienzle D, Silverstein DC, Chaffin K. Multiple myeloma in cats: variable presentation with different immunoglobulin isotypes in two cats. Vet Pathol 2000;37:364–9.

[75] Rusbridge C, Wheeler SJ, Lamb CR, et al. Vertebral plasma cell tumors in 8 dogs. J Vet Intern Med 1999;13:126–33.

[76] Berg J, Lamb CR, O'Callaghan MW. Bone scintigraphy in the initial evaluation of dogs with primary bone tumors. J Am Vet Med Assoc 1990;196:917–20.

[77] Thrall DE, LaRue SM. Palliative radiation therapy. Semin Vet Med Surg (Small Anim) 1995;10:205–8.

[78] Siegel S, Cronin KL. Palliative radiotherapy. Vet Clin North Am Small Anim Pract 1997;27:149–55.

[79] Vail DM, Powers BE, Getzy DM, et al. Evaluation of prognostic factors for dogs with synovial sarcoma: 36 cases (1986–1991). J Am Vet Med Assoc 1994;205:1300–7.

[80] Silva-Krott IU, Tucker RL, Meeks JC. Synovial sarcoma in a cat. J Am Vet Med Assoc 1993;203:1430–1.

[81] Fox DB, Cook JL, Kreeger JM, et al. Canine synovial sarcoma: a retrospective assessment of described prognostic criteria in 16 cases (1994–1999). J Am Anim Hosp Assoc 2002;38:347–55.

[82] Craig LE, Julian ME, Ferracone JD. The diagnosis and prognosis of synovial tumors in dogs: 35 cases. Vet Pathol 2002;39:66–73.

[83] Thamm DH, Mauldin EA, Edinger DT, et al. Primary osteosarcoma of the synovium in a dog. J Am Anim Hosp Assoc 2000;36:326–31.

[84] Lahmers SM, Mealey KL, Martinez SA, et al. Synovial T-cell lymphoma of the stifle in a dog. J Am Anim Hosp Assoc 2002;38:165–8.

[85] Meinkoth JH, Rochat MC, Cowell RL. Metastatic carcinoma presenting as hind-limb lameness: diagnosis by synovial fluid cytology. J Am Anim Hosp Assoc 1997;33:325–8.

[86] Hauck M. Feline injection site sarcomas. Vet Clin North Am Small Anim Pract 2003;33:553–7.

[87] Seguin B. Feline injection site sarcomas. Vet Clin North Am Small Anim Pract 2002;32:983–95.

[88] Hershey AE, Sorenmo KU, Hendrick MJ, et al. Prognosis for presumed feline vaccine-associated sarcoma after excision: 61 cases (1986–1996). J Am Vet Med Assoc 2000;216:58–61.

[89] Davidson EB, Gregory CR, Kass PH. Surgical excision of soft tissue fibrosarcomas in cats. Vet Surg 1997;26:265–9.

[90] Poirier VJ, Thamm DH, Kurzman ID, et al. Liposome-encapsulated doxorubicin (Doxil) and doxorubicin in the treatment of vaccine-associated sarcoma in cats. J Vet Intern Med 2002;16:726–31.

[91] Barber LG, Sorenmo KU, Cronin KL, et al. Combined doxorubicin and cyclophosphamide chemotherapy for nonresectable feline fibrosarcoma. J Am Anim Hosp Assoc 2000;36:416–21.

[92] Cronin K, Page RL, Spodnick G, et al. Radiation therapy and surgery for fibrosarcoma in 33 cats. Vet Radiol Ultrasound 1998;39:51–6.

[93] Bregazzi VS, LaRue SM, McNiel E, et al. Treatment with a combination of doxorubicin, surgery, and radiation versus surgery and radiation alone for cats with vaccine-associated sarcomas: 25 cases (1995–2000). J Am Vet Med Assoc 2001;218:547–50.

[94] Cohen M, Wright JC, Brawner WR, et al. Use of surgery and electron beam irradiation, with or without chemotherapy, for treatment of vaccine-associated sarcomas in cats: 78 cases (1996–2000). J Am Vet Med Assoc 2001;219:1582–9.

[95] Kobayashi T, Hauck ML, Dodge R, et al. Preoperative radiotherapy for vaccine associated sarcoma in 92 cats. Vet Radiol Ultrasound 2002;43:473–9.

[96] Vascellari M, Melchiotti E, Bozza MA, et al. Fibrosarcomas at presumed sites of injection in dogs: characteristics and comparison with non-vaccination site fibrosarcomas and feline post-vaccinal fibrosarcomas. J Vet Med A Physiol Pathol Clin Med 2003;50:286–91.

[97] Parchman MB, Crameri FM. Primary vertebral hemangiosarcoma in a dog. J Am Vet Med Assoc 1989;194:79–81.

[98] Levy MS, Kapatkin AS, Patnaik AK, et al. Spinal tumors in 37 dogs: clinical outcome and long-term survival (1987–1994). J Am Anim Hosp Assoc 1997;33(33):307–12.

[99] Jongeward SJ. Primary bone tumors. Vet Clin North Am Small Anim Pract 1985;15:609–41.

[100] Tucker DW, Olsen D, Kraft SL, et al. Primary hemangiosarcoma of the iliopsoas muscle eliciting a peripheral neuropathy. J Am Anim Hosp Assoc 2000;36:163–7.

[101] Ward H, Fox LE, Calderwood-Mays MB, et al. Cutaneous hemangiosarcoma in 25 dogs: a retrospective study. J Vet Intern Med 1994;8:345–8.

[102] Ogilvie GK, Powers BE, Mallinckrodt CH, et al. Surgery and doxorubicin in dogs with hemangiosarcoma. J Vet Intern Med 1996;10:379–84.

[103] Sorenmo KU, Baez JL, Clifford CA, et al. Efficacy and toxicity of a dose-intensified doxorubicin protocol in canine hemangiosarcoma. J Vet Intern Med 2004;18:209–13.

Vet Clin Small Anim 35 (2005) 1169–1194

VETERINARY CLINICS
SMALL ANIMAL PRACTICE

Traumatic Luxations of the Appendicular Skeleton

Jude T. Bordelon, DVM*, H. Fulton Reaugh, DVM,
Mark C. Rochat, DVM, MS

Department of Veterinary Clinical Sciences, College of Veterinary Medicine, Oklahoma State
University, 01 Farm Road, Stillwater, OK 74078, USA

Luxation, or dislocation, is usually defined as a separation of articulating joint surfaces. For the purposes of this discussion, luxation refers to the complete traumatic separation of opposing joint surfaces in conjunction with tearing of the associated joint capsule and one or more of the collateral ligaments or other supporting ligaments. The amount of energy necessary to disrupt the primary stabilizers of a joint (typically, the joint capsule and collateral ligaments) is substantial. As such, luxations are complex injuries that often result in concurrent damage to the articular cartilage, intra-articular structures (eg, menisci and cruciate ligaments), periarticular tendons and muscles, and, on occasion, neurovascular structures. Failure to identify the luxation and the extent of the injury promptly and accurately results in disruption of joint and limb mechanics, normal mechanisms for maintaining articular cartilage health, and further injury to the articular surface. Permanent cartilaginous injury, periarticular fibrosis, and loss of range of motion may occur if reduction and stabilization of the luxated joint do not occur in a timely fashion.

INITIAL ASSESSMENT

With any trauma, accurate and prompt assessment of the animal for all injuries is the initial goal. The proper diagnostic approach to trauma patients has been discussed elsewhere [1], but there are specific issues with regard to luxations that warrant discussion.

Because other regional injuries and swelling may obscure the presence of a luxation, dislocated joints may elude diagnosis during the initial examination of the acutely traumatized patient. Identification of a chronically luxated joint may be less complicated, but even under those circumstances, identifying a luxation of a joint surrounded by significant soft tissue (eg, the shoulder joint)

*Corresponding author. E-mail address: bjude@okstate.edu (J.T. Bordelon).

0195-5616/05/$ – see front matter
doi:10.1016/j.cvsm.2005.05.007

may be difficult. A thorough and more diligent examination should be performed for all joints in limbs in which swelling, abnormal limb shape or gait, pain, crepitus, or reluctance to bear weight is present.

Often, such an examination can only be accurately and humanely completed when the animal is heavily sedated or anesthetized. An animal's overall health status and ability to withstand anesthesia should be evaluated, at a minimum, by a complete blood cell count and serum biochemistry profile. Other diagnostic laboratory, radiographic, and electrodiagnostic methods, such as urinalysis, thoracic radiographs, and electrocardiography, are performed as indicated by the nature and timing of the injury [1].

During examination, careful palpation and manipulation of the joints is essential for diagnosis. Rarely is the diagnosis fully made through simple observation. It is best to develop a systematic approach to performing the orthopedic examination. The examination is begun at the distal extremities and progresses proximally. All joints should be palpated and manipulated to identify crepitus, pain, swelling (attributable to joint effusion, soft tissue edema, or hematoma), abnormal shape of the region of the limb around the joint, abnormal range of motion, and laxity. Any joint suspected of being luxated should be gently manipulated so as to avoid iatrogenic injury to the articular surfaces.

Confirmation of luxation is achieved by standard orthogonal radiographs. Radiographs also identify concurrent osteochondral or ligamentous avulsion fractures that may complicate management of the luxation. Other preexisting disorders that may prevent or reduce the chance of success of reduction techniques, such as hip dysplasia, Legg-Calvé-Perthes disease, and glenoid dysplasia, can also be identified. On occasion, oblique views may identify luxations not visualized on standard lateral and craniocaudal views. This is especially true for luxations of the digits and carpal bones. Similarly, stressed views may be necessary if standard radiographic evaluation fails to provide a diagnosis.

Finally, a word or two regarding the initial (temporary) management of luxations is appropriate. Once a luxation and other accompanying injuries or pre-existing conditions have been identified, the problem list must be prioritized and addressed accordingly (ie, life-threatening injuries take precedence over luxations). If other injuries or conditions preclude immediate correction of the luxation, the limb should be immobilized until definitive correction can be accomplished. For luxations at or below the elbow and stifle, a Robert Jones bandage or soft padded splint bandage should be applied [2]. Immobilizing the affected joint prevents further damage to articular and periarticular structures and minimizes pain associated with the unstable joint. For luxations of the shoulder and hip, a Spica bandage or Ehmer sling is more appropriate, because other bandages (Robert Jones or padded splint) cannot effectively immobilize these joints and, in fact, accentuate the instability and potential for further injury and pain by the pendulum effect created by the bandage [2].

MANAGEMENT OF SPECIFIC LUXATIONS

Digital luxation

Luxation of the digits (distal and proximal interphalangeal joints, carpometacarpal and tarsometatarsal joints) is a relatively common injury. Luxation of the distal interphalangeal joint is most common [3]. These luxations usually occur when the digit is restrained while the animal is in motion or when the digit is stepped on. The luxation usually presents with a varying but minimal degree of weight bearing that is accentuated by running or other activity. The digit may exhibit varying degrees of swelling, crepitus, and pain when palpated. Because of the multiangled and mobile nature of the digit of dogs and cats, diagnosis can be difficult. Careful palpation (with the aid of sedation, anesthesia, or digital nerve blockade [4] if overtly painful) of the extended joint may help the examiner to avoid interpreting normal rotation of the joint as joint instability. Standard radiographic projections may be of limited value, and oblique or stressed views may be necessary to diagnose the luxation. Osteoarticular and collateral ligament avulsion fractures may be observed on radiographs (Fig. 1).

Treatment options consist of primary repair of torn structures, digit amputation, arthrodesis, or external coaptation. Acute injuries, especially in working dogs, are best managed by primary repair of the torn joint capsule and associated collateral ligaments [3]. The nature of the foot requires careful preparation for surgery by precise clipping and scrubbing of all surfaces to reduce contamination. An adhesive iodine-impregnated barrier may also reduce contamination of the surgical site with resident bacterial flora. Intravenous antibiotics active against normal skin flora should also be administered

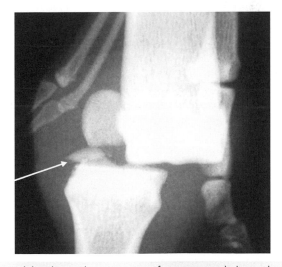

Fig. 1. Craniocaudal radiographic projection of a metatarsophalangeal joint dislocation in a kangaroo. Observe the articular avulsion fragment (*arrow*).

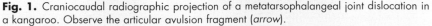

immediately before surgery, continued at 2- to 4-hour intervals during surgery, and continued in oral form for 5 to 7 days after surgery.

The incision is made directly over the affected aspect of the joint, and the torn joint capsule and collateral ligament are sutured with small, slowly absorbed, monofilament suture. A simple interrupted horizontal mattress or near-far-far-near pattern is most useful [3,4]. A single large mattress suture can be used to protect these sutures [3]. Because of the small, delicate, and complex nature of the anatomy of the digit, the use of a pneumatic tourniquet, fine-tipped instruments, magnification, and good lighting greatly improves the surgeon's ability to repair these delicate structures properly while decreasing the risk of iatrogenic damage to adjacent structures.

If a significant portion of the osteochondral surface of the luxated joint is fractured, anatomic reduction and lag screw fixation allow for primary bone healing to occur and limit the degree of secondary osteoarthritis [4]. Screw diameters as small as 1 mm are commercially available. With proper instrumentation and expertise, these fractures can be repaired with a high degree of success (Fig. 2). Even in the most skilled of hands, the ability to reduce and stabilize small fragments, such as those seen with collateral ligament rupture, properly is often impossible and usually unnecessary. If the fragment cannot be anatomically reduced and stabilized, it should be excised if it is located within the joint.

If primary repair of a torn collateral ligament is not possible, reconstruction of the collateral ligaments can be performed in one of two ways. With the first

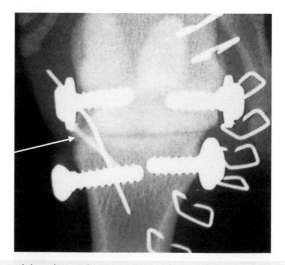

Fig. 2. Craniocaudal radiographic projection of the same metatarsophalangeal joint dislocation in a kangaroo after surgical reduction and stabilization. The collateral ligaments have been reconstructed with screws, washers, and nonabsorbable monofilament suture. The articular fragment has been anatomically reduced and secured with a 1-mm bone screw and 0.8-mm Kirschner wire (arrow).

method, the joint can be stabilized by placing small screws at the origin or insertion of the ligament. The screws are used as anchor points for nonabsorbable suture, such as polypropylene or polybutester, placed in a figure-of-eight pattern. The suture should be tied with the joint in extension and not overly tightened so as to prevent restriction of joint range of motion or varus or valgus deviation of the digit distal to the joint. The suture often loosens or breaks with time; therefore, its primary function is to maintain alignment for a period sufficient to allow functional fibrosis to occur.

Augmentation or replacement of collateral ligaments can be done using porcine small intestine submucosa. The submucosa, which is composed of several types of collagen, fibronectin, hyaluronic acid, heparin, heparin sulfate, chondroitin A, and growth factors [5], can then remodel into reparative tissue that closely resembles the original ligament [6]. One of the authors (MCR) has used this technique in a number of collateral ligament repairs in larger joints (Fig. 3), and although the results have been subjectively good, the true advantage of using submucosa as an alternative to suture remains unknown.

The second method of collateral ligament repair involves drilling a hole transversely across the respective metaphyses of the adjacent bones between the points of origin and insertion of the collateral ligaments. Nonabsorbable suture is then passed through the holes in a loop fashion such that a single suture passes through the hole, across the joint, through the other hole, and back across the joint. The suture is then tied with the joint in extension and with a mild amount of tension but not so tightly that the articular surfaces are compressed together. One disadvantage of this technique is that the entire repair is dependent on one suture and one knot. An advantage is that for joints with rupture of both collateral ligaments, the tendency for the joint to be deviated medially or laterally as one side is tied when using the anchor screw

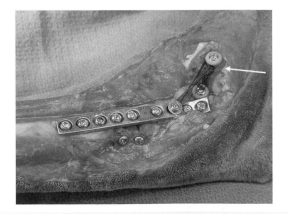

Fig. 3. Photograph of a hock shearing injury in a dog. The lateral collateral has been reconstructed with bone screws, washers, and porcine small intestine submucosa overlaid with monofilament nonabsorbable suture (*arrow*).

technique is avoided. In either technique, the anchor points, whether screws or holes, must be anatomically placed to avoid malalignment of the joint surfaces when the suture is tightened.

The limb is placed in a padded splint bandage for 2 to 3 weeks, followed by activity limited to walking for 2 weeks, with gradual return to full activity over the following 4 to 6 weeks. The prognosis for return to full function is good.

If the injury is chronic and the resulting fibroplasia or damage to articular structures prohibits definitive repair, arthrodesis of the joint can be performed for working or racing dogs with little loss of function. The general principles of arthrodesis include removal of articular cartilage, placement of autogenous cancellous bone graft in the arthrodesis site, and rigid fixation of the joint at a functional angle [7,8]. Small plates and screws generally work best for arthrodesis, but transarticular pinning is a reasonable alternative. External coaptation (padded splint) support is required until radiographic signs of osseous fusion are present (typically, 6–8 weeks). After removal of the splint, return to full function should occur over the next 3 to 4 weeks.

Amputation can also be performed for chronic luxations but is generally less preferred for the third and fourth digits because of their greater role in weight bearing compared with the second and fifth digits. Specific issues to consider when amputating a digit include removal of the palmar sesamoids when amputating the metacarpophalangeal joint, removal of the distal condyle of the proximal bone at the amputated joint, beveling the osteotomy when amputating the second and fifth metacarpophalangeal joints, and preserving the digital pad when amputating the interphalangeal joints [3].

Acute or chronic injuries in nonworking dogs can be managed by closed reduction and splinting of the affected limb for 3 to 4 weeks. When splinted, the joint capsule and collateral ligaments fibrose, allowing functional weight bearing and minimal pain. If the joint is chronically painful, arthrodesis or amputation, as discussed previously, is indicated.

Metacarpal and carpal luxation

Luxation of the carpometacarpal and middle carpal joints is uncommon and usually results from hyperextension injury. Although the many interconnecting carpal ligaments are usually disrupted, the loss of joint stability is primarily attributable to disruption of the palmar fibrocartilage. A complete discussion of carpal hyperextension injuries is beyond the scope of this article and has been previously discussed in detail [3,4,9]. These injuries are treated with partial or pancarpal arthrodesis, depending on the specific level and structures injured.

Antebrachiocarpal joint luxation is uncommon. Subluxation of the joint occurs with rupture of the radial or ulnar short collateral ligament, but true luxation can only occur when both are torn through the ligament or as an avulsion of the bony origin of the ligament [4]. Failure of the palmar structural supports also occurs, and carpal hyperextension and secondary osteoarthritis invariably occur. Reconstruction of the collaterals could be performed, but continued instability often leads to the need for pancarpal arthrodesis to allow use of the limb [4]. More common are partial subluxations resulting from shearing injuries of the carpus. The diagnosis and management of carpal shearing injuries have been discussed elsewhere [10–12].

Luxation of the radiocarpal bone is a rarely reported injury of dogs [3,4,13]. The luxation often occurs after a jump or fall that produces carpal hyperextension and pronation. This injury may be more common in Border Collies [13]. The force of impact ruptures the short radioulnar intercarpal ligaments, dorsal joint capsule, short ligaments between the radial carpal bone and the second and fourth carpal bones, short radial collateral ligament, and palmar radiocarpal and palmar ulnar carpal ligaments [4,13]. When radiocarpal bone luxation occurs, the radiocarpal bone is rotated 90° in a lateral-to-medial direction and in a dorsopalmar direction along the long axis of the bone. This leaves the radiocarpal bone positioned on the distopalmar surface of the radius. Concurrent fracture of the ulnar styloid or ulnar carpal bone has been reported [4]. The dog is commonly not weight bearing and holds the limb in abduction. The joint is swollen, painful, and held in an extended position. Palpation of the joint reveals a significant depression on the dorsal surface of the joint in the normal location of the radiocarpal bone, medial instability, and crepitus during range of motion [4,13]. The displaced bone may also be palpated on the medial palmar surface of the joint. Standard orthogonal radiographs confirm the diagnosis.

Treatment should not be delayed, because closed reduction soon after injury is possible in many cases. Medial carpal joint instability may require open reduction and surgical reconstruction of the short radial collateral ligament to achieve joint stability. A dorsal approach is made directly over the radial carpal bone, and a Kirschner wire is inserted into the radial carpal bone from the medial nonarticular side to facilitate reduction [13]. When reduction is achieved, the Kirschner wire is seated into the adjacent ulnar carpal bone to maintain reduction. Reconstruction of the short radial collateral ligament is achieved in the same manner as for digital collaterals, using screws or bone anchors to serve as anchor points for nonabsorbable suture placed in a figure-of-eight pattern. In larger dogs, the suture used for collateral ligament reconstruction can be secured to the radial styloid process using bone anchors, but in smaller dogs, small screws or a hole drilled cranial to caudal in the radial styloid process is recommended. The joint capsule is then sutured. The limb is immobilized in slight flexion for 4 to 6 weeks, followed by gradual reduction in the degree of splint rigidity, increasing extension of the carpus, and slow return to normal activity. The prognosis for return to function is good after open reduction and reconstruction of the joint. Pancarpal arthrodesis is indicated if the radiocarpal bone cannot be reduced (usually because of chronicity) or when concurrent unreconstructable ulnar carpal bone fractures are present.

Chronic luxations or any type of carpal luxation that is persistently unstable or painful can be arthrodesed [3,4]. The basic principles of arthrodesis are followed as described previously. Angles for arthrodesis have been reported [8]. If the antebrachiocarpal joint is intact, partial carpal arthrodesis of the intercarpal and carpometacarpal joints is indicated, but involvement of the antebrachiocarpal joint requires pancarpal arthrodesis for long-term successful limb use [14]. Cranial pancarpal arthrodesis plate and screw application is preferred for pancarpal arthrodesis. For partial carpal arthrodesis, a T-plate and screws are the preferred method of fixation, although some authors report the use of cross-pinning techniques in smaller dogs [4].

Elbow luxation

Intrinsic stability of the elbow is afforded by the rigid congruity of the anconeus, olecranon fossa, and humeral epicondyles during the ground phase of the animal's gait when the joint is in extension. Additionally, all three bones of the elbow are connected by the medial and lateral collateral ligaments. The collateral ligaments provide primary ligamentous support for the elbow [15]. The oblique ligament, the olecranon ligament, and the annular ligament also provide secondary support for the elbow. The orientation of the oblique and olecranon ligaments also imparts an inherent medial stability as compared with the lateral aspect of the joint.

Traumatic luxation of the elbow joint invariably occurs in a lateral direction because of the more rounded lateral epicondyle and the larger and squarer medial epicondyle (Fig. 4). Valgus bending and indirect rotational forces also contribute to the high percentage of lateral luxations [16–18]. Further, the lateral collateral ligament is stronger than the medial collateral ligament, which

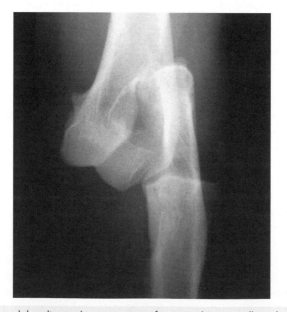

Fig. 4. Craniocaudal radiographic projection of a typical canine elbow luxation with the radius and ulna luxated lateral to the humeral condyle.

may allow the medial collateral ligament to fail first when the joint is traumatized. Luxation usually occurs when the elbow is flexed beyond 90°, preventing the humeral epicondyles from restraining the anconeal process.

Elbow luxation is commonly presented as a non–weight-bearing lameness, with abduction and supination of the limb and an irregular lateral contour of the elbow and mild flexion [16,17]. Pain, decreased range of motion, and crepitus are also evident on manipulation of the elbow. As many as 50% of elbow luxations may have rupture of the lateral and medial collateral ligaments [16]. Collateral instability can be assessed by flexing the elbow and carpus 90° and rotating the carpus in a clockwise or counterclockwise direction. Normal medial collateral ligament integrity allows the carpus to be internally rotated (pronated) 60°, whereas normal external rotation (supination) of the carpus is approximately 40° [16]. On occasion, the flexor and extensor muscles of the antebrachium may also be avulsed from their origins on the ulna and humerus. Radiographs are taken to identify concurrent fractures. It is common to see small avulsion fractures of the lateral collateral ligament, but the bony fragment is rarely of sufficient size to require surgical stabilization or excision.

If significant fractures are not present, closed reduction should be performed immediately while the animal is still anesthetized for radiographs. Studies have demonstrated no advantage of open reduction over closed reduction if the joint is stable after reduction [19–21]. The elbow is reduced by flexing the joint greater than 90° and, while maintaining flexion, inwardly rotating and adducting the distal limb to allow the anconeal process to engage the lateral epicondyle. With lateral digital pressure, continued pronation, and slow extension, the anconeal process is reduced into the olecranon fossa medial to the lateral epicondyle [16–21]. A deep plane of anesthesia, brachial plexus blockade with local anesthetics, and even nondepolarizing muscle relaxants can all be used to allow sufficient muscle relaxation to achieve reduction [16–18]. If the reduced elbow is palpably stable, the limb is placed in a Spica splint with the elbow moderately extended at an angle of approximately 140° for a period of 5 to 7 days, followed by daily gentle passive range-of-motion exercises and controlled weight bearing for 2 to 4 weeks [17,18]. Nonsteroidal anti-inflammatory drugs are administered for analgesia. If the luxation is reduced in a closed fashion but is subjectively more unstable, the Spica splint is maintained for 2 weeks and range-of-motion exercises and limited weight bearing are then performed for 3 to 4 weeks [18].

If the luxation cannot be reduced or if gross instability is present after closed reduction, open reduction should be performed [16–18]. A caudolateral surgical approach is used for most luxations, but reconstruction of the medial collateral ligament requires a separate medial approach. Reduction of the luxation is performed in the same manner as for a closed reduction if possible. If the bones are grossly overridden and muscle contracture is severe, a blunt periosteal elevator can be used to lever the ulna and radius into reduction, but extreme caution should be taken to avoid damaging the articular surfaces of the joint [16–18]. Extremely difficult reductions can be facilitated by the use of a fracture distractor [16]. Temporary fixation pins are placed in the distal humerus and proximal ulna, and the distractor is used to spread the bone surfaces apart mechanically and gain reduction. Because of the extreme mechanical advantage this device affords, caution should be taken to avoid iatrogenic tearing of muscles and ligaments and overstretching of neuro-vascular bundles [16].

The lateral collateral ligament often requires reconstruction, augmentation, or primary repair to achieve joint stability. Primary repair of a torn collateral ligament is accomplished by reapposing the ligament edges if the tear occurs midligament or by the use of a bone anchor or screw to reattach a ligament avulsed from its origin or insertion. Monofilament nonabsorbable suture material and tension-sparing suture patterns, such as a locking loop pattern, are used in either scenario. If the collateral ligament cannot be primarily repaired, reconstruction or augmentation is achieved in the same manner as for digital collaterals using screws or bone anchors and nonabsorbable suture or fiber wire. The personal experience of one of the authors (MCR) suggests that braided suture materials may be more prone to fraying and premature failure than monofilament suture. The postoperative management of elbow luxations is the same as with closed reduction except that the Spica splint is maintained for 3 weeks before beginning physical therapy. The prognosis for elbow luxation is good to excellent for return to full function if closed reduction or early surgical treatment is performed. If treatment is delayed or the damage to the intra- and periarticular structures is significant, a less favorable outcome may result.

Chronic luxations or luxations that are persistently unstable can be arthrodesed [22,23]. The basic principles of arthrodesis are followed as described previously. Angles for arthrodesis have been reported [8], and caudal plate and screw application is the fixation method of choice. An emerging alternative to arthrodesis is total elbow arthroplasty [24]. This is a technically demanding procedure currently performed on a limited basis but one that may hold promise for restoring elbow function.

Shoulder luxation

The scapulohumeral or shoulder joint is primarily a ball and socket joint. Primary restraint of the joint is provided by the collateral ligaments and the joint capsule [25,26]. Secondary support is provided by the supraspinatus, subscapularis, infraspinatus, and teres minor muscles [25]. Luxation of the shoulder is an uncommon traumatic event in dogs and rarely occurs in cats. Although shoulder luxation can occur in any direction, lateral displacement most commonly occurs as a result of combinations of extreme adduction, flexion, and supination [25]. Clinical signs of shoulder luxation include non–weight-bearing lameness, flexion of the joint, and pain with manipulation of the limb. Lateral luxation results in notable prominence of the greater tubercle, lateral displacement of the tubercle with respect to the acromion and spine of the scapula, and internal rotation of the foot. With medial luxation, the tubercle is medial to its normal location and the foot is externally rotated. Range of motion of the shoulder is limited and painful. The dermatomes of the brachial plexus should be evaluated to identify concurrent peripheral neurologic injury [27]. Because intrathoracic injuries often occur concomitantly with thoracic limb injuries, thoracic radiographs and an electrocardiogram are indicated before administering general anesthesia [28]. Examination of the shoulder under anesthesia demonstrates malalignment and crepitus of the joint. Even under normal circumstances, the humerus can usually be abducted much more than might be expected; thus, a diagnosis of medial shoulder instability or luxation should be made with caution if based on degree of abduction alone. Orthogonal radiographs should demonstrate the luxation, and any accompanying fractures of the glenoid, acromion, or proximal humerus should be identified. Fractures other than small fragments associated with collateral ligaments should be surgically addressed.

Closed reduction is often possible under heavy sedation or general anesthesia if no significant fractures are present and the luxation is acute. For a lateral luxation, the humerus is tractioned distally and lateral pressure is applied to the humeral head while medial pressure is applied to the scapula with the opposite hand. If closed reduction of a lateral luxation is successful and the joint is stable, the limb is immobilized in a Spica splint or non–weight-bearing sling for 2 to 3 weeks to maintain the humeral head in the glenoid. A medial luxation is reduced by simultaneous distal traction and application of medial pressure to the humeral head while applying lateral pressure to the scapula. After successful reduction, the limb is maintained in a Velpeau bandage for 2 to 3 weeks. Radiographs are made after reduction and stabilization to confirm proper reduction.

Surgical reduction and stabilization are indicated when the luxation cannot be reduced or when gross instability remains. Historically, the preferred method of surgical stabilization of medial and lateral luxations has vacillated between reconstruction of the collateral ligaments and medial or lateral transposition of the biceps brachii tendon. Although effective, biceps brachii tendon transposition alters the biomechanics of the shoulder [25]. Radiographic and histologic examination of transposed biceps tendons reveals osteoarthritis, tearing of the midsubstance of the tendon, and joint incongruency [25]. Although dogs seem to adapt to the changes that result from biceps tendon transfer, reconstruction of the affected glenohumeral ligaments with non-absorbable suture and bone screws or anchors is considered the preferred treatment [29]. Although more technically demanding, this technique affords shoulder stability without compromising function of the biceps brachii tendon and joint biomechanics [29].

The limb is usually maintained in a non–weight-bearing sling for 2 weeks, followed by passive range-of-motion exercises and leash-controlled weight bearing on nonslick surfaces for 4 weeks. Return to full activity is then allowed to occur over the following 4 weeks if no instability or complications are encountered. Chronic shoulder luxations may require operative intervention because of excessive periarticular fibrosis. If the degree of fibrosis, loss of range of motion, or damage to articular structures is judged to be excessive, arthrodesis of the shoulder or glenoid excision arthroplasty may be considered as a salvage technique. Arthrodesis of the shoulder may result in more consistent and better results in small dogs [25,30] but is an appropriate option for large dogs. Glenoid excision arthroplasty may offer a good to excellent prognosis in dogs [31]. The usefulness of this procedure in medium to large breeds or patients with concurrent orthopedic disease remains unclear at this time. The authors prefer to perform glenoid excision as described by Franczuszki and Parkes [31], leaving the humeral head intact.

Hip luxation

The hip is the most commonly luxated joint in the dog and cat. Hip luxation usually occurs unilaterally but occurs bilaterally in a small percentage of cases [32]. The hip is stabilized primarily by the ligament of the head of the femur, the joint capsule, and the dorsal acetabular rim [32]. Secondary stabilizers include the labrum, the ventral acetabular ligament, and the muscles the surrounding the hip [32]. The direction of luxation is almost always craniodorsal secondary to external rotation and adduction of the limb [32–35]. Ventral luxation is the second most common direction for luxation but is considerably less common [33]. Luxation in other directions, in the experience of the authors, usually represents significant injury to the periarticular soft tissue structures of the hip, and the femoral head is free to move in any direction. Craniodorsal luxations result in a characteristic externally rotated and adducted limb carriage. The limb length is shortened when compared with the opposite limb. Animals with hip luxation are typically minimally weight bearing or non-weight bearing if the luxation is acute but can become weight bearing with chronicity. Ventral luxations are usually internally rotated, and the greater trochanter is displaced medially [33].

When the hip is normal, drawing an imaginary line between the greater trochanter, ischiatic tuberosity, and craniodorsal iliac crest creates a shallow "V" shape [35]. When the hip is luxated craniodorsally, the greater trochanter lies along a line drawn between the iliac crest and ischiatic tuberosity. Gentle manipulation of the hip often reveals crepitus, decreased range of motion, and pain. External rotation of the femur while placing the examiner's opposite thumb in the depression between the greater trochanter and ischiatic tuberosity results in expulsion of the thumb from the depression in the normal hip. When the hip is luxated craniodorsally, the femoral head cannot pivot about the acetabulum and the femur fails to dislodge the examiner's thumb (known as a negative thumb test) [35]. Although these findings are highly suggestive of a hip luxation, other hip pathologic findings can be present. Orthogonal radiographs are always indicated with suspected hip luxation to identify concurrent fractures of the greater trochanter, femoral neck, capital physis, or acetabulum; avulsion fractures of the ligament of the head of the femur; and concurrent degenerative conditions, such as hip dysplasia and Legg-Calvés-Perthes disease [32,33,35].

If no concurrent pathologic findings exist, closed reduction is appropriate. Although closed reduction typically becomes more difficult when luxation has been present for more than 4 to 5 days, closed reduction should be attempted before open reduction in all cases if no contraindications to closed reduction (ie, ligament of the head of the femur avulsion fracture or other fractures) are present. If closed and stable reduction is possible, the negative aspects of surgery are avoided. The caveat to this approach is that the likelihood of successful reduction decreases considerably under these circumstances, and client communication and preparation for surgery should be addressed ahead of time so that operative intervention can be directly pursued while the animal is still anesthetized.

Closed reduction is performed with the animal under general anesthesia. Administration of epidural analgesia or anesthetic further relaxes the pelvic musculature, facilitates reduction, and provides pain relief after reduction. The animal can be placed on its back and the limb suspended to elevate the pelvis slightly from the table for several minutes to relax the pelvic musculature further [32,33,35]. To perform the reduction, the animal is positioned in lateral recumbency and a thin but nonabrasive sling (eg, folded towel) is passed around the inguinal region of the limb and held by an assistant standing behind the animal. The person performing the reduction maneuver stands opposite the assistant and grasps the distal limb. The limb is tractioned distally and externally rotated. This positions the femoral head on the craniodorsal rim of the acetabulum. With continued distal traction and lateral pressure on the greater trochanter, the hip is internally rotated to reduce the femoral head into the acetabulum. If a definitive "pop" or "clunk" is heard, the limb is circumducted while maintaining pressure on the greater trochanter to push hematoma and residual joint capsule or other soft tissue out of the acetabulum. The thumb test can then be gently performed (while avoiding external rotation and extension) to assess the relative degree of stability of the reduced hip [32]. If the hip is palpably reduced and stable, the limb is placed in a modified Ehmer sling. The goal of the modified Ehmer sling is to create internal rotation and abduction to stabilize the hip maximally while fibrosis of the joint capsule occurs. The original Ehmer sling does not have a band placed around the caudal abdomen; only the limb is wrapped from thigh to foot. This approach would seemingly have little effect on the hip joint above the tape. Passing a tape strip from the foot to an abdominal band (modified Ehmer sling) does create some degree of internal rotation and abduction. Modified Ehmer slings are difficult to apply properly; even when correctly applied, they can result in significant soft tissue abrasion and vascular compromise. It is critical that the owner be advised of the potential for serious complications and the sling be examined by the veterinarian every 3 to 4 days to identify problems before significant damage occurs [32,33,35]. Any potential problem with a modified Ehmer sling observed by an owner should be immediately investigated so as to avoid serious complications, including loss of the limb. Closed reduction of a hip luxation is usually successful approximately 35% to 50% of the time

[32,33]. Cats generally do not tolerate Ehmer slings and may need to be tranquilized for a brief period [32]. If the hip remains stable after 7 to 10 days, the limb can cautiously be allowed to bear weight to a limited degree or the limb can be placed in a Robinson sling for an additional 2 weeks. Exercise restriction is continued for 6 to 8 weeks after removal of the sling. Fewer complications typically occur with a Robinson sling than with a modified Ehmer sling, and the Robinson sling allows movement of the hip joint. Joint motion helps to decrease adhesions, increases polysulfated glycosaminoglycan and hyaluronic acid synthesis in the joint, improves the orderly arrangement of reparative collagen deposition, and increases the rate of clearance of hematoma from the joint space [32].

Closed reduction of ventral luxations involves general and epidural anesthesia as previously discussed. The femur is tractioned distally and laterally to reduce the femoral head into the acetabulum [32,33,35]. A modified Ehmer sling should not be applied, because abduction of the limb can luxate the hip. Hobbles can be placed on the animal's pelvic limbs, but in one of the authors' experience (MCR), the reduced hip is relatively stable and the animal can usually be managed with strict cage confinement for 2 to 3 weeks.

Grossly unstable hips, hips with concurrent pathologic findings or preexisting disease that may prevent stable reduction, or hips that cannot be reduced should be repaired by operative methods. In addition to general anesthesia, epidural anesthesia facilitates reduction and reduces postoperative pain. Numerous techniques for stabilization of a luxated hip have been described [32,33,35–38]. A common misconception about operative treatment of craniodorsal hip luxations is that one method is appropriate for all situations. The specific reasons why closed reduction cannot be achieved are usually unknown before surgery. Sometimes, the mere presence of an infolded edematous joint capsule in the acetabulum is all that prevents reduction, whereas in other cases, significant injury to the joint capsule and surrounding soft tissues is present. Therefore, the joint should be approached by a craniolateral approach, and the extent of the injury should be assessed. The craniolateral approach can be easily converted to a trochanteric osteotomy if such is required for visualization and repair of the luxation. If only the joint capsule or excess ligament of the head of the femur impedes reduction, the offending structures are removed from the acetabulum, the hip is reduced, a capsulorrhaphy is performed, and the hip is gently externally rotated to test for stability. If adequate stability is present, the remainder of the incision is closed and the animal is confined to a small cage or the limb is placed in a Robinson or modified Ehmer sling depending on the preference of the surgeon. By definition, rupture of the ligament of the head of the femur must occur for the femoral head to luxate from the acetabulum. The ligament, because of its location and nature, cannot be primarily repaired. If the other primary stabilizers of the hip, joint capsule, and acetabular labrum have been damaged beyond primary repair, other methods to achieve joint stability can be used. Often, if the nature of the luxation requires the use of these techniques, the surgical approach should be converted to a greater trochanteric osteotomy so as to allow exposure to perform these techniques properly. If the trochanter is osteotomized, it should be reattached caudal and distal to the osteotomy line to stretch the gluteal muscles over the dorsal aspect of the hip and provide an additional but temporary stabilizing force to the repair [33,35]. Methods for stabilizing the hip include dorsal augmentation with suture secured to the acetabular rim with bone screws or anchors, Knowles toggle pinning or other techniques for creating neoligament of the head of the femur, transacetabular pinning, suture augmentation from the cranial aspect of the acetabulum to the base of the femoral neck, dynamic transarticular pinning, caudodistal translocation of the greater trochanter, and ilioischial (deVita) pinning [32,33,35–40]. Ilioischial pinning can also be performed in conjunction with closed reduction but cannot be done in cats, because the straight nature of the feline pelvis does not allow the pin to anchor in the iliac wing or ventral to the ischiatic tuberosity. Of these techniques, the authors prefer the Knowles toggle pinning and dorsal suture augmentation techniques. In the interest of brevity, the specific technical details of these techniques are described elsewhere [32,33,35–40]. Dogs with hip luxation and concurrent hip dysplasia without secondary changes can be managed by performing a triple pelvic osteotomy in conjunction with definitive repair of the luxation [41]. One of the most difficult scenarios to address is the luxated hip that is complicated by hip dysplasia or Legg-Calvés-Perthes disease and the secondary osteoarthritis. Dogs affected with hip luxation and concurrent Legg-Calvés-Perthes disease are small dogs and, as such, can be effectively managed with excision arthroplasty if reduction, closed or open, is unsuccessful. Larger dogs with hip dysplasia and secondary osteoarthritis can sometimes be successfully managed with closed or open reduction techniques, but the owner must be made aware of the decreased potential for success. Alternative techniques for treating hip luxation under these circumstances include excision arthroplasty (femoral head and neck excision) and total hip arthroplasty. The decision to proceed with hip excision arthroplasty or total hip replacement should be made before attempting reduction in the event that stable reduction cannot be achieved. Most experts agree that total hip arthroplasty results in better function than excision arthroplasty for large dogs but necessitates extra presurgical preparation for the possibility that conversion of an open reduction attempt to a total hip replacement is required. Arthrodesis of the hip is not possible, because fusion of the joint prohibits the entire pelvic limb from being advanced.

Other concurrent injuries associated with the luxation, such as avulsion fragments from the ligament of the head of the femur, acetabular fractures, capital physeal fractures, and femoral neck fractures, are addressed as recommended elsewhere [33].

How an individual animal is managed after open reduction depends on the degree of stability achieved by the repair, the nature of the animal, and the compliance of the owner. Postoperative management can range from weight bearing and cage confinement for a period of 3 to 8 weeks to placement of non–weight-bearing slings for a similar period. If the damage to the articular surface is minimal and stable reduction is achieved, the prognosis is generally good for return to normal function [42]. The prognosis for hip luxations managed with salvage procedures (excision or total hip arthroplasty) is also generally good to excellent with proper technique, patient selection, and absence of complications.

Patellar luxation

Traumatic luxation of the patella is an uncommon occurrence [43]. It is a distinctly different disorder from the far more common congenital patellar luxation. Traumatic patellar luxation results from a direct blow to the craniomedial or craniolateral stifle that disrupts the soft tissue constraints of the femoropatellar joint, often referred to as the retinaculum. The bony anatomy and overall limb alignment, unlike those of dogs with congenital luxations, are normal. The limb is held in flexion and internally rotated if a medial luxation has occurred or externally rotated in the instance of lateral patellar luxation [43]. Varying degrees of pain, swelling, and loss of range of motion occur. Radiographs and orthopedic examination while the animal is sedated may be necessary to identify the luxated patella because of the associated swelling and displacement of the patella from its normal location in the trochlear sulcus.

A standard parapatellar approach is made on the side that is injured. The patella is reduced, and the torn retinaculum is sutured with monofilament absorbable or nonabsorbable suture in an interrupted tension-sparing pattern. If the soft tissue–supporting structures are accurately apposed, the patellofemoral articulation is generally stable throughout a range of motion. If elements of patellar luxation are present that, with injury, encourage continued patellar luxation, other components of patellar luxation repair (ie, wedge or rectangle recession trochleoplasty, desmotomy, tibial crest translocation) should be performed [43–45]. The repair is supported by a padded splint bandage for 2 weeks, followed by an additional 2 to 4 weeks of activity limited to brief walks on a leash. The prognosis is generally good.

Stifle luxation

Luxation of the stifle is uncommon and is often referred to as stifle derangement. Stifle derangement is more common in cats than in dogs [43,44]. Stifle luxation is a disruption of most, if not all, of the ligamentous restraints of the stifle [43–48]. Disruption of both cruciate ligaments and at least one of the collateral ligaments is the most common scenario. Primary stabilization of the stifle is provided by the paired cruciate ligaments and paired collateral ligaments. Additional support is provided by the tendon of the long digital extensor muscle, tendon of the popliteus muscle, patellar tendon, menisci, and joint capsule [44].

The diagnosis of stifle derangement is made primarily by palpation [43–48]. Individual tests used to identify isolated injuries of the stifle (eg, cranial drawer sign for cranial cruciate ligament rupture) can be difficult to perform and evaluate because of the gross instability present in stifle derangement. General anesthesia or heavy sedation is usually necessary for proper evaluation. Varus and valgus instabilities are best evaluated with the stifle rotationally aligned and extended [44]. Cruciate ligament injuries are evaluated with the stifle rotationally aligned and partially flexed. Care should be taken to ensure that cranial or caudal drawer maneuvers are begun with the stifle in a neutral position.

Neurovascular injuries are uncommon, but forces significant enough to produce stifle derangement may also damage the popliteal artery and the saphenous, tibial, and peroneal nerves [43]. The limb distal to the stifle should be assessed for peripheral nerve function by nociception within defined dermatomes [27]. Vascular integrity can be assessed by palpation of the dorsal pedal artery at the hock or by Doppler detection methods (Fig. 5). Nuclear scintigraphy is not logistically prudent in the acutely traumatized patient. Angiography is not commonly performed in veterinary medicine, making the procedure often inefficient, time-consuming, and excessively complicated.

Radiographs are useful for identifying avulsion injuries of the cruciate and collateral ligaments and concurrent osteochondral fractures. Stress views are often necessary to demonstrate collateral ligament injuries (Fig. 6). Surgical exploration is usually necessary to determine the full extent of the soft tissue injuries. Nonbony avulsions, midsubstance tears, and injuries to the small tendons of the stifle (long digital extensor and popliteus tendon) can best be identified and properly evaluated by surgical methods. Likewise, although the patellar tendon is rarely avulsed, tears of the supporting fascia and patellofabellar ligaments are common. If these supporting elements are ruptured, patellar luxation (medial, lateral, or gross instability) may be present.

Treatment of stifle derangement by external coaptation or transarticular pinning has reportedly been successful in small dogs and cats [43,44,47]. Pin migration can occur, and return of full function may not occur. Extra-articular

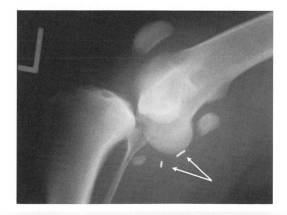

Fig. 5. Lateral radiographic projection of a luxated stifle with concurrent injury to branches of the popliteal artery. Hemoclips were used to achieve hemostasis of the injured vessels (*arrows*).

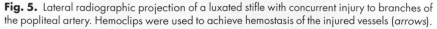

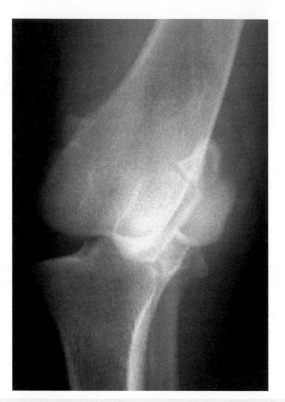

Fig. 6. Craniocaudal radiographic projection of a luxated stifle with a medial force being applied to demonstrate ligamentous disruption.

suture techniques, augmented by placement of a transarticular external skeletal fixator, have been reported to produce satisfactory results as well [43]. The goal of all these techniques is to provide temporary stabilization that allows for the development and maturation of sufficient fibrous tissue to maintain joint orientation and functional range of motion.

A more precise approach is surgical reconstruction or augmentation of each specific anatomic structure that is damaged. Surgical exploration can be accomplished through a medial or lateral parapatellar approach depending on which stifle components are injured. Meniscal injuries are debrided if irreparable, but only the damaged portion of the meniscus should be removed to maintain as much meniscal function as possible [45]. If meniscal separation from the medial or lateral joint margins is present but the meniscus is intact, the meniscus should be sutured in situ using small monofilament nonabsorbable or slowly absorbed suture [46].

Treatment of osteochondral fragments depends on the size of the fragment. Reattachment by the use of positional or lag screws or diverging Kirschner wires should be performed if the fragment is large enough to allow reattachment. Screw heads and Kirschner wires should be seated flush with the surface of the cartilage. Full-thickness cartilage injuries should curetted or foraged to enhance development of reparative fibrocartilage [49].

Collateral ligament injuries can be repaired by ligamentorrhaphy if a distinct tear occurs with viable ligament on either side of the tear. If bony avulsion occurs, diverging Kirschner wires, a screw and spike plate combination, or a screw and washer combination can be used to reattach the avulsed segment of bone. If the ligament is avulsed from the bone, suture anchors or bone screws can be employed for reattachment. Augmentation is performed when the ligament is stretched or partially torn. Creation of a new ligament is performed when the ligament is disrupted to the point where no primary repair can be accomplished. Whether augmentation or recreation is needed, screws can be combined with nonabsorbable suture, prosthetic meshes (eg, polypropylene), or xenograft materials (eg, porcine small intestine submucosa) to create a neoligament that is eventually supported by fibrous tissue. It is important to place the origin and insertion points of any repair in the exact anatomic location of the original ligament and not to place excessive tension on the repair so as to avoid creating forces that result in abnormal spatial relations between the femur and tibia. Abnormal alignment in any plane seems to set the stage for failure of the repair or may create abnormal loading and movement of the joint, resulting in pain and dysfunction.

Injuries to the cranial and caudal cruciate ligaments can be addressed by any number of extra- and intracapsular techniques, each with their advantages and disadvantages. Extracapsular techniques, such as the DeAngelis or fibular head transposition (FHT) technique, may create abnormal rotational malalignment or, in the case of the FHT, be impossible to perform if the lateral collateral ligament is damaged. Techniques that provide more symmetry, such as the Piermattei and Flo [43] or Schwarz encircling technique, may be more applicable, but care should be taken to avoid overtightening the suture(s) supplanting the cranial cruciate ligament, because excessive tension can create caudal translocation of the tibia if the caudal cruciate ligament is ruptured. The applicability of the tibial plateau leveling osteotomy (TPLO) procedure to the deranged stifle is unknown but may be an appropriate option. Overrotation should be diligently avoided to prevent excessive strain on an intact caudal cruciate ligament or the creation of caudal drawer in the event that the caudal cruciate ligament is ruptured during the injury.

Intracapsular techniques using autogenous or allograft materials can also be performed, but, again, excessive tensioning of the graft replacing the cranial or caudal cruciate ligament can result in malalignment of the femorotibial compartment, abnormal loading and wear, and pain.

Popliteal or long digital extensor tendon avulsion can be repaired in the same manner as collateral ligament disruptions. Care should be taken not to place implants in the joint that project excessively above the joint surface. Testing of range of motion of the joint should be performed while directly observing the implant to determine if impingement by the implant on corresponding anatomic structures occurs. The tendon of the long digital extensor muscle can also be transfixed to the proximal tibia if insufficient length or excessive tension is present when anatomic repositioning is attempted. Injuries to the patellar support ligaments or fascia are sutured in apposition after reduction of the patella and repair of other intra-articular structures. Excessive tension should be avoided so as to prevent creating a luxation on the side of the injury.

After anatomic reconstruction, the repair is supported by external coaptation for at least 2 weeks. If the patient and client are amenable to physical therapy and facilities for such are available, recent work supports the implementation of physical therapy early in the rehabilitation course [50,51]. Two weeks after surgery, the dog should begin daily controlled passive range-of-motion exercises to preserve extension, alternated with swimming or water treadmill exercises to encourage full flexion [50]. Joint motion helps to decrease adhesions, increases polysulfated glycosaminoglycan and hyaluronic acid synthesis in the joint, improves the orderly arrangement of reparative collagen deposition, and increases the rate of clearance of hematoma from the joint space.

The use of nonsteroidal anti-inflammatory drugs and heat and cold therapy lessens pain associated with physical therapy, enhances blood flow to the joint, and facilitates physical therapy. Chondroprotectants, such as chondroitin sulfate/glucosamine combinations and polysulfated glycosaminoglycans, may improve the intra-articular environment and enhance the reparative process.

If extensive damage is present or the stifle is chronically unstable and painful, amputation or arthrodesis is a viable option. Generally, midfemoral amputation results in better overall function than stifle arthrodesis. The prognosis for return to normal nonathletic function is surprisingly good if stability and normal alignment can be achieved [43–45]. The likelihood of returning to full athletic function is less likely, because osteoarthritis and some loss of range of motion occur.

Hock luxation

Luxation of the hock, or talocrural joint, is a somewhat common event [52–54]. Generally, the medial or lateral collateral ligament is ruptured, but simultaneous rupture or avulsion of the medial and lateral collateral ligaments is rare. Shearing injuries are common and result in varying degrees of loss of a collateral ligament (usually, the lateral collateral ligament) and subluxation of the joint. As with the carpus, shearing injuries are a distinct type of injury that has been discussed elsewhere in great detail [55,56].

If a ligamentous injury sufficient to allow luxation of the joint occurs, the diagnosis is generally straightforward and is made largely by physical examination findings. Malalignment, loss of range of motion, and pain are present when the joint is examined. Fracture of the distal tibia (classically, Salter-Harris type 1) may appear similar, but standard orthogonal radiographic views readily provide the diagnosis. Management of hock luxations is aimed at reconstruction of the affected collateral ligament [52–54]. If the ligament has been avulsed form the bone, reattachment using bone screws or suture anchors and nonabsorbable monofilament suture in a tension-sparing pattern is appropriate. Generally, the relatively flat collateral ligament is most accurately and easily apposed with a locking loop or modified Krackow pattern. Short and long components of the collaterals should be inspected and repaired individually as needed [54]. Fracture of a significant portion of the tibial or fibular malleolus can also allow luxation to occur (Fig. 7). Because both malleoli contribute to the shape of the tibial mortise and articular surface of the joint, accurate reduction and rigid fixation are important to minimize joint instability and osteoarthritis. Depending on the fracture and bone configuration, the fragment can be secured with lag screws or Kirschner wires and a tension band wire (Fig. 8). Application of a splint after surgery protects the repair and promotes unimpeded fracture healing but does set the stage for joint fibrosis and loss of range of motion. The use of a hinged transarticular fixator may offer protection to the surgical repair while preserving more joint range of motion.

The prognosis for luxation of the hock not associated with shearing injury is generally good for nonperformance dogs if anatomic reduction and stabilization can be performed in a timely manner. Racing dogs generally do not return to full athletic performance [57].

Luxation of the individual bones of the tarsus occurs rarely [52,54,57]. Subluxation of the tarsal joints is more common. Luxation or subluxation often occurs in conjunction with fracture of one or more of the tarsal bones. Much like the carpus, the small bones of the tarsus are stabilized by multiple interconnecting ligaments. Rupture of the ligaments is required for luxation to occur. Primary repair of the ligaments is impossible, and fibrosis by splinting is generally unrewarding. For those reasons, surgical fusion of the affected bone and adjacent bones is usually the best course of action.

Animals with tarsal bone luxation generally present with varying degrees of swelling, pain, and reluctance to use the limb. Palpation of the affected area may reveal a deformity or incongruency. Orthogonal radiographs generally demonstrate the luxation, but oblique views are occasionally required to visualize the luxation and associated fractures. Depending on the extent and specific location of the luxation, the involved joints are arthrodesed using standard principles of arthrodesis and bone screws are placed in lag fashion [58,59]. Small bone plates and screws or screws and a figure-of-eight wire are used for tarsometatarsal, calcaneoquartal, centrodistal, and talocentral luxations.

Because of the tremendous distractive forces placed on the calcaneus by the common calcaneal tendon, luxation of this bone usually requires the application of a bone plate laterally or an intramedullary pin and plantar tension band wire to achieve uncomplicated arthrodesis of the calcaneoquartal and calcaneotalar joints [52,57].

The surgical repair is protected by a padded caudal splint for 4 to 6 weeks, followed by gradual return to full activity over the following 4 to 6 weeks. The prognosis for return to full activity is usually good.

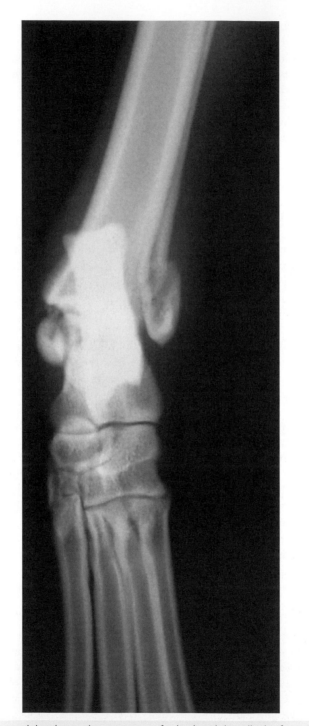

Fig. 7. Craniocaudal radiographic projection of a hock with bimalleolar fractures.

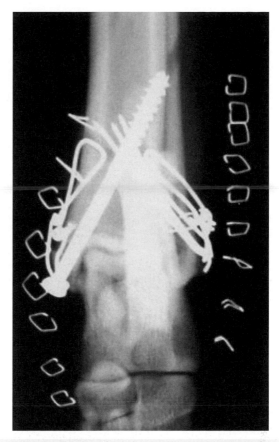

Fig. 8. Craniocaudal radiographic projection of a hock with bimalleolar fractures after surgical reduction and stabilization of the fractures with a cannulated screw and figure-of-eight tension band (medial malleolus) and Kirschner wires and a figure-of-eight tension band (lateral malleolus).

Metatarsal and digital luxation

Tarsometatarsal, metatarsophalangeal, and digital luxations are managed in the same manner as the corresponding joints of the thoracic limb.

References

[1] Rochat MC. Considerations for successful fracture repair. Vet Med (Praha) 2001;96:375–84.

[2] DeCamp CE. External coaptation. In: Slatter D, editor. Textbook of small animal surgery. 3rd edition. Philadelphia: WB Saunders; 2003. p. 1838–41.

[3] Piermattei DL, Flo GL. Fractures and other conditions of the carpus, metacarpus, and phalanges. In: Handbook of small animal orthopedics and fracture repair. Philadelphia: WB Saunders; 1997. p. 344–89.

[4] Eaton-Wells RD. Injuries of the digits and pads. In: Bloomberg MS, Dee JF, Taylor RA, editors. Canine sports medicine and surgery. 1st edition. Philadelphia: WB Saunders; 1998. p. 165–73.

[5] Badylak SF. SIS fact sheet. In: Proceedings of the Third SIS Symposium. 2000. p. 2.

[6] Musahl V, Abramowitch SD, Gilbert TW, et al. The use of porcine small intestinal submucosa to enhance the healing of the medial collateral ligament—a functional tissue engineering study in rabbits. Orthop Res 2004;22(1):214–20.

[7] Rochat MC, Mann FA. Metatarsophalangeal arthrodesis in three dogs. J Am Anim Hosp Assoc 1998;34:158–63.

[8] Watson C, Rochat M, Payton M. Effect of weight bearing on the joint angles of the fore- and hind limb of the dog. Vet Comp Orthop Traumatol 2003;16:250–4.

[9] Johnson AL, Hulse DA. Carpal luxation and subluxation. In: Fossum TW, editor. Small animal surgery. 2nd edition. St. Louis Missouri: Mosby; 2002. p. 1089–92.

[10] Probst CW, Millis DL. Carpus and digits. In: Slatter D, editor. Textbook of small animal surgery. 3rd edition. Philadelphia: WB Saunders; 2003. p. 1974–88.

[11] Van Gundy T. Carpal shearing injuries: algorithm and treatment. In: Bojrab MJ, Ellison GW, Slocum B, editors. Current techniques in small animal surgery. 4th edition. Philadelphia: Williams & Wilkins; 1998. p. 114–6.

[12] Benson JA, Boudrieau RJ. Severe carpal and tarsal shearing injuries treated with an immediate arthrodesis in seven dogs. J Am Anim Hosp Assoc 2002;38:370–80.

[13] Miller A, Carmichael S, Anderson TJ, et al. Luxation of the radial carpal bone in four dogs. J Small Anim Pract 1990;31:148–54.

[14] Early T. Canine carpal ligament injuries. Vet Clin North Am Small Anim Pract 1978;8:183–99.

[15] Vogelsang RL, Vasseur PB, Peauroi JR, et al. Structural, material, and anatomic characteristics of the collateral ligaments of the canine cubital joint. Am J Vet Res 1997;58:461–6.

[16] Dassler C, Vasseur PB. Elbow luxation. In: Slatter D, editor. Textbook of small animal surgery. 3rd edition. Philadelphia: WB Saunders; 2003. p. 1919–27.

[17] Piermattei DL, Flo GL. The elbow joint. In: Handbook of small animal orthopedics and fracture repair. Philadelphia: WB Saunders; 1997. p. 288–320.

[18] Johnson AL, Hulse DA. Traumatic elbow luxation. In: Fossum TW, editor. Small animal surgery. 2nd edition. St. Louis, MO: Mosby; 2002. p. 1079–84.

[19] Schaeffer IGF, Wolvekamp P, Meij BP, et al. Traumatic luxation of the elbow in 31 dogs. Vet Comp Orthop Traumatol 1999;12:33–9.

[20] O'Brien MG, Boudrieau RJ, Clark GN. Traumatic luxation of the cubital joint (elbow) in dogs: 44 cases (1978–1988). J Am Vet Med Assoc 1992;201(11):1760–5.

[21] Billings LA, Vasseur PB, Todoroff RJ, et al. Clinical results after reduction of traumatic elbow luxations in nine dogs and one cat. J Am Anim Hosp Assoc 1992;28:137–42.

[22] Moak PC, Lewis DD, Roe SC, et al. Arthrodesis of the elbow in three cats. Vet Comp Orthop Traumatol 2000;13:149–53.

[23] de Haan JJ, Roe SC, Lewis DD, et al. Elbow arthrodesis in twelve dogs. Vet Comp Orthop Traumatol 1996;9:115–8.

[24] Conzemius MG, Aper RL, Corti LB. Short-term outcome after total elbow arthroplasty in dogs with severe, naturally occurring osteoarthritis. J Am Vet Med Assoc 2003;32:545–52.

[25] Talcott KW, Vasseur PB. Luxation of the scapulohumeral joint. In: Slatter D, editor. Textbook of small animal surgery. 3rd edition. Philadelphia: WB Saunders; 2003. p. 1897–904.

[26] Piermattei DL, Flo GL. The shoulder joint. In: Handbook of small animal orthopedics and fracture repair. Philadelphia: WB Saunders; 1997. p. 228–60.

[27] Oliver JE, Lorenz MD, Kornegay JN. Neurologic history and examination. In: Handbook of veterinary neurology. 3rd edition. Philadelphia: WB Saunders; 1997. p. 3–46.

[28] Houlton JEF, Dyce J. Does fracture pattern influence thoracic trauma? Vet Comp Orthop Traumatol 1992;5:90–2.

[29] Fitch RB, Breshears L, Staatz A, et al. Clinical evaluation of prosthetic medial glenohumeral ligament repair in the dog (ten cases). Vet Comp Orthop Traumatol 2001;14:222–8.

[30] Fowler JD, Presnell KR, Holmberg DL. Scapulohumeral arthrodesis: results in seven dogs. J Am Anim Hosp Assoc 1988;24:667–72.

[31] Franczuszki D, Parkes LJ. Glenoid excision as a treatment in chronic shoulder disabilities: surgical technique and clinical results. J Am Anim Hosp Assoc 1988;24:637–43.

[32] Holsworth IG, DeCamp CE. Coxofemoral luxation. In: Slatter D, editor. Textbook of small animal surgery. 3rd edition. Philadelphia: WB Saunders; 2003. p. 2002–8.

[33] Piermattei DL, Flo GL. The hip joint. In: Handbook of small animal orthopedics and fracture repair. Philadelphia: WB Saunders; 1997. p. 422–68.

[34] Wadsworth PL. Biomechanics of luxations. In: Bojrab MJ, editor. Disease mechanisms in small animal surgery. 2nd edition. Philadelphia: Lea & Febiger; 1993. p. 1048–59.

[35] Johnson AL, Hulse DA. Coxofemoral luxation. In: Fossum TW, editor. Small animal surgery. 2nd edition. St. Louis, MO: Mosby; 2002. p. 1102–9.

[36] Mehl NB. A new method of surgical treatment of hip dislocation in dogs and cats. J Small Anim Pract 1988;29:789–95.

[37] Beckham HP, Smith MM, Kern DA. Use of a modified toggle pin for repair of coxofemoral luxation in dogs with multiple orthopedic injuries: 14 cases (1986–1994). J Am Vet Med Assoc 1996;208(1):81–4.

[38] Özaydin I, Kiliç E, Baran V, et al. Reduction and stabilization of hip laxity by the transposition of the ligamentum sacrotuberale in dogs: an in vivo study. Vet Surg 2003;32:46–51.

[39] McLaughlin RM, Tillson DM. Flexible external fixation for craniodorsal coxofemoral luxations in dogs. Vet Surg 1994;23:21–30.

[40] Beale BS, Lewis DD, Parker RB, et al. Ischio-ilial pinning for stabilization of coxofemoral luxations in twenty-one dogs: a retrospective evaluation. Vet Comp Orthop Traumatol 1991;4:28–34.

[41] Murphy ST, Lewis DD, Kerwin SC. Traumatic coxofemoral luxation in dysplastic dogs managed with a triple pelvic osteotomy: results in four dogs. Vet Comp Orthop Traumatol 1997;10:136–40.

[42] Evers P, Johnston GR, Wallace LJ, et al. Long-term results of treatment of traumatic coxofemoral joint dislocation in dogs: 64 cases (1973–1992). J Am Vet Med Assoc 1997;210(1):59–64.

[43] Piermattei DL, Flo GL. The stifle joint. In: Handbook of small animal orthopedics and fracture repair. Philadelphia: WB Saunders; 1997. p. 516–80.

[44] Vasseur PB. Stifle joint. In: Slatter D, editor. Textbook of small animal surgery. 3rd edition. Philadelphia: WB Saunders; 2003. p. 2090–133.

[45] Johnson AL, Hulse DA. Medial and lateral patellar luxation. In: Fossum TW, editor. Small animal surgery. 2nd edition. St. Louis, MO: Mosby; 2002. p. 1133–42.

[46] Bruce WJ. Multiple ligamentous injuries of the canine stifle joint: a study of 12 cases. J Small Anim Pract 1998;39:333–40.

[47] Welches CD, Scavelli TD. Transarticular pinning to repair luxation of the stifle joint in dogs and cats: a retrospective study of 10 cases. J Am Anim Hosp Assoc 1990;26:207–14.

[48] Hulse DA, Shires P. Multiple ligament injury of the stifle joint in the dog. J Am Anim Hosp Assoc 1986;22:105–10.

[49] Rudd RG, Visco DM, Kincaid SA, et al. The effects of beveling the margins of articular cartilage defects in immature dogs. Vet Surg 1987;16(5):378–83.

[50] Marsolais GS, Dvorak G, Conzemius MG. Effects of postoperative rehabilitation on limb function after cranial cruciate ligament surgery in the dog. J Am Vet Med Assoc 2002;220:1325–30.

[51] Marsolais GS, McLean S, Derrick T, et al. Kinematic analysis of the hind limb during swimming and walking in healthy dogs and dogs with surgically corrected cranial cruciate ligament rupture. J Am Vet Med Assoc 2003;222:739–43.

[52] Welch JA. The tarsus and metatarsus. In: Slatter D, editor. Textbook of small animal surgery. 3rd edition. Philadelphia: WB Saunders; 2003. p. 2158–69.

[53] Johnson AL, Hulse DA. Ligament injury of the tarsus. In: Fossum TW, editor. Small animal surgery. 2nd edition. St. Louis, MO: Mosby; 2002. p. 1143–50.

[54] Piermattei DL, Flo GL. Fractures and other orthopedic injuries of the tarsus, metatarsus, and phalanges. In: Handbook of small animal orthopedics and fracture repair. Philadelphia: WB Saunders; 1997. p. 607–55.

[55] Diamond DW, Besso J, Boudrieau RJ. Evaluation of joint stabilization for treatment of shearing injuries of the tarsus in 20 dogs. J Am Anim Hosp Assoc 1999;35(2):47–53.

[56] Beardsley SL, Schrader SC. Treatment of dogs with wounds of the limbs caused by shearing forces: 98 cases (1975–1993). J Am Vet Med Assoc 1995;207(8):1071–5.

[57] Dee JF. Tarsal injuries. In: Bloomberg MS, Dee JF, Taylor RA, editors. Canine sports medicine and surgery. 1st edition. Philadelphia: WB Saunders; 1998. p. 120–37.

[58] Fettig AA, McCarthy RJ, Kowaleski MP. Intertarsal and tarsometatarsal arthrodesis using 2.0/2.7-mm or 2.7/3.5-mm hybrid dynamic compression plates. J Am Anim Hosp Assoc 2002;38:364–9.

[59] Wilke VL, Robinson TM, Dueland RT. Intertarsal and tarsometatarsal arthrodesis using a plantar approach. Vet Comp Orthop Traumatol 2000;13:28–33.

Vet Clin Small Anim 35 (2005) 1195–1211

VETERINARY CLINICS
SMALL ANIMAL PRACTICE

Healing, Diagnosis, Repair, and Rehabilitation of Tendon Conditions

Maria A. Fahie, DVM, MS

College of Veterinary Medicine, Western University of Health Sciences,
309 East Second Street, Pomona, CA 91766, USA

Information regarding the epidemiologic significance of canine and feline patients clinically affected by tendon conditions is not readily available in the veterinary literature. Despite that, the conditions are clinically relevant, and management can be frustrating because of difficulty with diagnosis, choice of treatment or repair technique, prolonged tissue healing, and potential for permanent compromise of limb function after surgery. This article reviews tendon healing and reported tendon conditions, focusing on bicipital tenosynovitis and common calcaneal tendon (CCT) injuries. Surgical management options, research in enhancement of tendon healing, and postoperative rehabilitation are also reviewed.

TENDON HEALING
Anatomy
Tendons are composed of tenocytes, which produce an extracellular matrix of collagen, elastin, proteoglycans, glycoproteins, and primarily type I collagen fibers generally running parallel to the long axis of the tendon. The tensile strength of tendon is similar to that of bone and is usually greater than ordinary demands of activity. The gliding function of the tendon is facilitated by its continuous arrangement of epitenon, paratenon, and endotenon. The epitenon is the superficial connective tissue sheath of a tendon. The paratenon is loose areolar tissue within the substance of the tendon. The endotenon is composed of type III collagen fibers that facilitate innervation and vascular supply because they form smaller separate tendon fascicles.

Tendon sheaths act to reduce friction in locations in which there is marked change in tendon direction. They have an inner visceral layer that is closely attached to the tendon by areolar tissue and an outer parietal layer that is attached to adjacent connective tissue or periosteum. The two layers arc connected by the mesotendon, which is also important for innervation and vascular supply of ensheathed tendons [1].

E-mail address: mfahie@westernu.edu

0195-5616/05/$ – see front matter
doi:10.1016/j.cvsm.2005.05.008

Tendons are classified as vascular and avascular. Vascular tendons, such as the deep gluteal tendon, have improved healing and receive blood supply from vessels within surrounding muscle, periosteum, and connective tissue. Avascular tendons, such as the biceps tendon, are surrounded by a tendon sheath with a synovial membrane lining and synovial fluid. Some intrinsic vessels enter the tendon sheath for a short distance, and others originate from the mesotendon, resulting in neovascularization of the paratenon and tendon core [2].

Clinical significance

The goal of surgical repair of tendon injury in small animal patients is primarily to restore adequate tensile strength to support weight bearing. Maintenance of gliding function is a secondary goal in small animal patients because of their lack of digital dexterity compared with human beings [1]. Because vascular supply is relatively sparse, precautions are indicated to reduce tissue trauma during surgery and to prevent excessive postoperative weight bearing. The mechanisms of restoration of tendon strength are not completely understood and are likely complex multifactorial processes [3]. There are two main theories supported by experimental evidence in the human literature: extrinsic and intrinsic healing. With extrinsic healing, the tendon is believed to have no internal healing ability and relies on formation of adhesions, infiltration of inflammatory cells and fibroblasts, and extratendinous vascular supply. Intrinsic healing is believed to rely on proliferation of epitenon and endotenon with intratendinous vascular supply and no adhesion formation [4].

Wound healing occurs in the same stages as in other soft connective tissues, and minimizing gap formation between damaged tendon ends is optimal [5]. A large gap results in increased scar tissue primarily composed of type III collagen, which is more elastic than the normal type 1 collagen in uninjured tendon [6]. Fibroblasts from the epitenon, paratenon, and surrounding areolar tissue produce collagen. Collagen production within a damaged tendon peaks between 5 and 12 days after injury, has a lesser rate of increase from 12 to 21 days, and is then markedly lower to day 60. Tensile strength increases by 16 days after injury because of collagen fiber cross-linking and reorientation [7]. Conflicting resources exist regarding the issue of postoperative immobilization. Complete limb immobilization, such as with a transarticular external fixator, for longer than 21 days resulted in a significant reduction in vascularity at the wound site [8]. Less vigorous external coaptation, such as a cranial or caudal splint, could be recommended for at least an additional 21 days to promote collagen orientation that is parallel to tendon stress [9,10]. Some research in human patients supports the concept of limited immediate mobilization to enhance restoration of the gliding mechanism, which results in a stronger and more histologically normal repair compared with immobilized tendon [11].

TENDON CONDITIONS OF THE THORACIC LIMB

Thoracic limb lameness is a common problem in young and adult patients. A simple diagnosis of osteoarthritis of the glenohumeral joint based on radiographic changes warrants further diagnostic exploration. Tendon conditions, including bicipital tears or tenosynovitis and supraspinatus calcification, are increasingly diagnosed as specific causes of lameness primarily because of the expanding availability of and experience with arthroscopic exploration of the glenohumeral joint [12,13]. The biceps brachii tendon may also play a role in medial shoulder instability syndrome [14,15]. Additional reported traumatic injuries include triceps tendon avulsion and superficial and deep digital flexor tendon laceration [16]. Thorough orthopedic examination is indicated for localization of the potential source of lameness. Orthopedic examination of the shoulder is described in the section on bicipital tenosynovitis diagnosis in this article.

Classification of biceps tendon lesions

Two studies report classification schemes for biceps tendon lesions, one based on ultrasonographic findings and one based on arthroscopic findings. Biceps tenosynovitis is ranked by increasing severity (grades 1–4) of pathologic changes in the tendon and tendon sheath, which were visualized ultrasonographically in a study of 120 dogs [17]. Pathologic changes included an anechoic ring around the tendon, loss of tendon homogenicity, and a hyperechoic border of the tendon sheath. The following disease processes of the biceps tendon were diagnosed with ultrasound in that study: tenosynovitis, corpora libera in the tendon sheath (caused by osteochondritis dissecans), exostoses of the intertubercular groove (sulcus), partial and complete tendon rupture, fractured supraglenoid tubercle, scar formation (indicative of an old injury), luxation, and tumor and hematoma within the tendon sheath [17].

Six subtypes of biceps tendon lesions were classified arthroscopically in 23 dogs and a cat: 1. complete or partial avulsion, tear from the supraglenoid tubercle, 2. midsubstance tear, 3. tendinitis, 4. bipartite tendon, 5. luxation, and 6. tenosynovitis [18].

BICIPITAL TENOSYNOVITIS

Bicipital tenosynovitis is an inflammation of the intracapsular extrasynovial region of the tendon of the biceps brachii muscle within the intertubercular groove. Affected dogs have a history of intermittent or progressive weight-bearing thoracic limb lameness that worsens with activity. The cause is direct or indirect trauma to the tendon or tendon sheath. Direct trauma includes repetitive injury, and indirect trauma can result from proliferative fibrous connective tissue, osteophytes, adhesions between the tendon and sheath, or mineralization of the supraspinatus tendon [19]. The condition affects primarily medium- to large-breed middle-aged dogs [18,20]. The right shoulder was affected almost twice as often as the left in a study of 29 dogs [20], perhaps because of a dominant thoracic limb as in human beings. Pathologic findings include synovial proliferation, edema, fibrosis, and lymphocytic-plasmacytic infiltration of the tendon and synovium [20]. Dystrophic mineralization and cartilaginous metaplasia of the biceps tendon are also reported [20,21].

Diagnosis

Diagnosis of bicipital tenosynovitis is controversial and often a diagnosis of exclusion, based primarily on history; orthopedic examination findings; synovial fluid cytology; and imaging studies, such as radiographs, ultrasonography, magnetic resonance imaging, computed tomography, and arthroscopy. Arthroscopy plays a dual role as a diagnostic and therapeutic tool; therefore, it may be the most cost-effective option.

Orthopedic examination of the shoulder joint should include range of motion with hyperflexion and hyperextension, a biceps tendon test, and assessment of joint stability or shoulder drawer. The biceps tendon test involves palpation of the tendon within the intertubercular groove while the joint is fully extended. Shoulder drawer is performed similarly to stifle drawer. The scapula is held with the thumb on the acromion and the index finger wrapped around the craniomedial side of the scapular neck. The humerus is held with the other hand, with the thumb on the caudolateral proximal humeral metaphysis and index finger on the greater tubercle. The shoulder joint should be partially flexed and tested cranially, caudally, medially, and laterally for palpable translocation. A grading system of shoulder drawer laxity has been reported with grade 1 (no translocation), grade 2 (mild, humeral head motion palpable), grade 3 (moderate, able to move the humeral head onto the rim of glenoid cavity), and grade 4 (severe, dislocated). Palpation comparison with the contralateral limb is warranted [14].

Typical orthopedic examination findings in cases of bicipital tenosynovitis include a positive biceps tendon test with pain on palpation of the biceps tendon within the intertubercular groove and on shoulder hyperextension. Supraspinatus and infraspinatus muscle atrophy may be evident. Synovial fluid analysis is consistent with degenerative joint disease and is nonspecific [20].

Radiographic evaluation of the shoulder should require anesthesia and include mediolateral and craniocaudal views, with stressed mediolateral views if shoulder instability is suspected [14]. Radiographic views to highlight the intertubercular groove are recommended and include the flexed craniodistal-cranioproximal view. The dog can be placed in dorsal recumbency with the affected shoulder hyperflexed and the limb rotated laterally. Arthrography may identify filling defects along the biceps tendon [20].

In cases of bicipital tenosynovitis, radiographs may reveal intertubercular groove osteophytes and sclerosis, osteophytes on the caudal aspect of the humeral head or the caudal aspect of the glenoid rim, and mineralization of the biceps tendon (Fig. 1) [20]. Radiographic changes in the intertubercular groove region are not necessarily associated with clinical signs of lameness, however [17].

High-frequency (at least 7.5–10 MHz) linear transducers are recommended to visualize the biceps tendon ultrasonographically, and the technique was reported to be more sensitive and less invasive than arthrography in one study [17] but less sensitive in another study [22]. Findings typical of bicipital tenosynovitis include a hypoechoic to anechoic area surrounding the tendon with mild to severe tendon thickening [17].

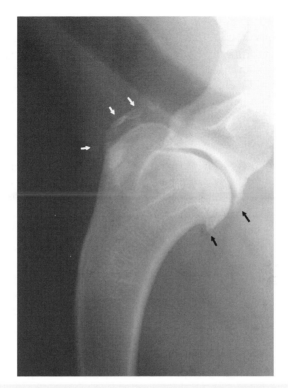

Fig. 1. Radiograph of shoulder with bicipital tenosynovitis. (*From* Burk RL, Feeney DA. Small animal radiology and ultrasonography. A diagnostic text and atlas. 3rd edition. Philadelphia: WB Saunders; 2003. p. 590; with permission.)

Medical management

Literature regarding the success of medical management of bicipital tenosynovitis is sparse. Results reported in one study [20] revealed excellent to good results in 7 of 17 patients returned for clinical assessment at a mean of 5 months after treatment. Administration of methylprednisolone acetate at a dose of 10 to 40 mg into the biceps tendon and tendon sheath was performed at intervals of up to every 2 weeks and at a frequency from one to three times. Exercise restriction was recommended for 2 weeks after each injection.

Surgical management

Bicipital tenosynovitis is reported to be surgically managed via tenotomy (with or without tenodesis) and tenolysis. Tenodesis involves severing the tendon at its origin on the scapular supraglenoid tubercle and reattaching it to the lateral aspect of the proximal humerus [23,24]. Literature regarding the success of biceps brachii tenodesis is sparse, and assessment is complicated by variations in surgical technique and postoperative rehabilitation protocols. In one study, however, all dogs having postoperative clinical assessment had excellent (8 of

12 dogs) or good (4 of 12 dogs) results, with the ability to return to pre-diagnosis function [20].

Tenolysis means freeing a tendon from surrounding adhesions, and tenotomy means surgical incision of the tendon. In cases of bicipital tenosynovitis, both techniques involve transection of the tendon without reattachment, allowing it to drop down toward the humerus, where it becomes fixed with scar tissue [19,25,26]. Arthroscopic surgery enables debridement of hyperplastic synovium and tendon combined with tenolysis [19]. Supraspinatus tendon transection can additionally be performed if abnormalities are identified. The postoperative prognosis for cases of bicipital tenosynovitis managed arthroscopically is reported to depend on the degree of pathologic change, with most animals experiencing pain relief and restoration of good to excellent function within 4 to 8 weeks [19].

Recently, two minimally invasive tenolysis techniques (palpation guided and ultrasound guided) were compared and presented as potentially viable alternatives to arthroscopic tenolysis [27].

A standard methodology for assessment of the shoulder would enhance the ability to collect and report evidence-based results to assist with future therapeutic choices. Such a protocol has been proposed [28]. Research that may positively affect management of bicipital tenosynovitis is discussed in the section on enhancement of tendon healing later in this article.

TENDON CONDITIONS OF THE PELVIC LIMB

With the exception of superficial digital flexor displacement, tendon problems in the pelvic limb are generally traumatic, including lacerations of the patellar tendon; laceration or avulsion of the CCT or one of its components, such as the gastrocnemius tendon; and laceration of the superficial or deep digital flexor tendons. Superficial digital flexor displacement is a rare condition, which is apparently overrepresented in Shetland Sheepdogs, with primarily lateral displacement of the tendon as it passes over the tuber calcanei [29]. Surgical reconstruction of the disrupted soft tissue structures is recommended, and there was a return to normal function in nine of nine reported cases [29].

The literature specifically regarding patellar tendon laceration and repair is sparse, consisting primarily of case reports and a textbook chapter [15,30,31]. One case report describes repair using fascia lata autografts augmented with bone tunnels and monofilament nylon [30]. A similar augmentation technique was used with primary repair in three dogs [31]. The textbook chapter describes primary tendon apposition and repair for acute injuries and tendon lengthening techniques for chronic injuries [15].

COMMON CALCANEAN (ACHILLES) TENDON INJURIES

The CCT consists of three structures: the gastrocnemius tendon; the superficial digital flexor tendon; and the common tendon of the gracilis, biceps femoris, and semitendinosus muscles. All three attach to the calcaneal tuber of the fibular tarsal bone (calcaneus).

Classification of common calcaneal tendon lesions

A classification system has been proposed based on the anatomic location and gross pathologic findings of CCT lesions [32]. Type 1 is a complete rupture. Type 2 has three subtypes for partial rupture with a lengthened CCT system: A indicates musculotendinous rupture, B indicates CCT rupture with an intact paratenon, and C indicates gastrocnemius tendon avulsion with an intact superficial digital flexor tendon. Type 3 is tendinosis or peritendinitis.

Diagnosis

A thorough history and orthopedic examination are indicated in all cases. Orthopedic examination of patients with CCT injuries can reveal information regarding the severity of the injury. Patients with type 1 complete CCT rupture have a plantigrade stance on the affected limb with weight bearing. On palpation with the stifle fully extended, the tibiotarsal joint can be completely flexed without flexor tension of the digits. In acute cases, the tendon ends may be palpable. In chronic cases, they may be atrophied. Patients with type 2A partial musculotendinous injuries have a greater degree of hock flexion than in the contralateral normal limb. Patients with type 2C gastrocnemius tendon avulsion injuries can have striking digital flexion while standing, and digital flexural contracture is marked on palpation (Fig. 2). Patients with type 3 tendinosis or peritendinitis injuries have a normal stance with no ability to flex the hock when the stifle is fully extended [33]. Type 3 lesions are briefly described but may progress to type 2C lesions [32]. Bilateral lesions of all types are possible, and the associated gait or stance must be distinguished from

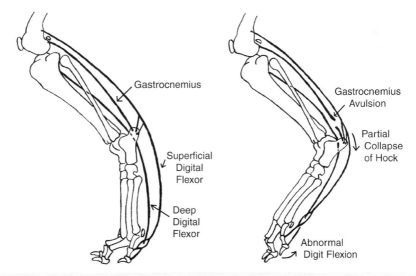

Fig. 2. (*Left*) Normal tendon anatomy during weight bearing. (*Right*) Type 2C gastrocnemius tendon avulsion with intact superficial digital flexor tendon demonstrates the mechanism of abnormal digital flexion during weight bearing.

neurologic or neuromuscular conditions, which should have normal palpation and inability to flex the hock with the stifle fully extended.

Conservative management
Conservative management without surgical anastomosis is controversial. The gap at the site of the injured tendon fills with scar tissue, possibly impairing function and predisposing the tendon to reinjury [1]. A large retrospective study in human beings concluded that surgical management was associated with lower risk of rerupture but higher risk of other complications, including infection, adhesions, and disturbed skin sensitivity [34].

SURGICAL MANAGEMENT
Surgical management of patellar tendon, CCT, and superficial or deep digital flexor tendon injuries is recommended and consists of primary apposition of ruptured tendon ends and temporary immobilization of the associated joint. A number of suture patterns and immobilization methods have been reported and are summarized in the following sections.

Primary versus secondary repair
Primary repair involves immediate apposition of tendon ends and can be performed in wounds that are minimally contaminated and well debrided [1,7]. More complicated wounds associated with fractures or having compromised tissue viability should have appropriate wound management, associated joint immobilization, and secondary tendon repair 2 to 4 weeks later [1,7]. The practice of secondary tendon repair is discouraged in human patients because of the associated loss of gliding function. In veterinary patients, however, the primary goal of surgical repair is restoration of tendon length for support. The degree of debridement of scar tissue at the site of secondary tendon repair or chronic tendon injury is controversial but recommended to be minimal in case reports [33,35].

Suture material and size
The ideal tendon suture material is nonreactive with high tensile strength and knot stability. The author's preference includes nonabsorbable suture materials, such as nylon, polypropylene, or polybutester. Some authors recommend nylon, stainless steel, polydioxanone, or polyglyconate, with a guideline of 3-0 to 0 United States Pharmacopeia (USP) sizes [1,36]. A study of human hand flexor tendons compared the same suture pattern (locking loop) with three different suture sizes (2-0, 3-0, and 4-0) and found that the pattern was strongest with 2-0 suture [37]. A 1986 study comparing the strength of two suture patterns in dogs used no. 2 braided polyester fiber [38]. A study of Achilles reconstruction in four dogs used 3-0 polydioxanone, and two studies of canine and goat tendon suture pattern comparisons used 2-0 polypropylene [39–41]. The tendency to use larger suture material could deleteriously affect healing because of the increased foreign body reaction.

Tendon anastomosis

Techniques for tendon anastomosis include many reported suture patterns. Choice of suture pattern is an important factor in tendon healing. The ideal suture pattern provides tensile strength and resistance to gap formation at the anastomosis site and minimally affects tendon vascular supply. This section summarizes the literature available for the following suture patterns: Bunnell-Mayer, Mason-Allen, simple interrupted (Fig. 3), locking loop (modified Kessler), double locking loop, three-loop pulley (Fig. 4), Krackow, continuous cruciate, and far-near-near-far (Fig. 5).

A 1989 study comparing the Bunnell-Mayer, modified Kessler, Mason-Allen, and simple interrupted patterns in goat superficial digital flexor and extensor tendons determined that the Bunnell pattern caused severe tendon constriction and the Mason-Allen and simple interrupted patterns pulled out, causing tendon laceration [41]. The modified Kessler pattern was concluded to be the best pattern in that study because of its balance of adequate tensile strength and relatively minimal tissue compromise.

Currently, several tendon suture patterns are recommended in the veterinary literature: locking loop (modified Kessler), double locking loop, three-loop pulley, Krackow, continuous cruciate, and far-near-near-far. The literature depicts three versions of a locking loop, varied by location of the suture knot. In one source, the knot is within the anastomosis site, and two other sources depict the knot as external to the anastomosis site laterally or on the midline of the tendon [1,37,41].

The double locking loop is described with the suture knot location external and lateral to the anastomosis site [40]. The double locking loop results in four

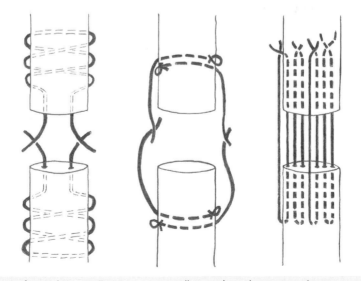

Fig. 3. (*Left to right*) Bunnell-Mayer, Mason-Allen, and simple interrupted suture patterns.

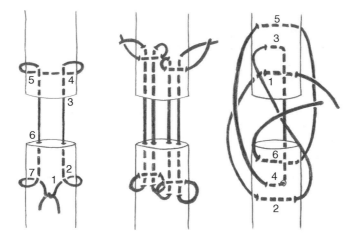

Fig. 4. (*Left to right*) Locking loop (modified Kessler), double locking loop, and three-loop pulley suture patterns.

strands of suture crossing the anastomosis site and was proven to be significantly stronger than the locking loop with only two strands [42].

Comparison of the three-loop pulley and locking loop patterns reveal the three-loop pulley to have the greater tensile strength with minimal gap formation in the triceps tendon [38]. The three-loop pulley is best applied to round tendons because of its three-dimensional configuration. It is more resistant to gap formation and faster to place than two locking loop sutures in the Achilles tendon [40].

The Krackow suture pattern is a Ford interlocking pattern on each edge of the tendon, and variations in suture placement were recently studied in rabbit

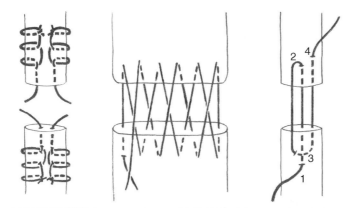

Fig. 5. (*Left to right*) Krackow, continuous cruciate, and far-near-near-far suture patterns.

Achilles tendon [15,43]. There was no significant strength difference when sutures were placed 0.5 cm apart versus 1 cm apart.

The continuous cruciate pattern was found to have increased strength characteristics when compared with the locking loop pattern in the relatively flat deep gluteal tendon [44]. The locking loop pattern had increased strength when compared with the Krackow pattern in the relatively flat patellar tendon [45]. The far-near-near-far suture is also suggested for flat tendons, but no biomechanical testing results were identified [46].

Closure of the epitenon (tendon sheath) is controversial because of the issue of adhesion formation. It can be performed using simple interrupted or simple continuous sutures [1]. Another reference discourages closure of the tendon sheath and recommends removal of the fibrous sheath at the anastomosis site [7].

The veterinarian should be familiar with tendon anastomosis choices, advantages, and disadvantages so as to make the appropriate decision on an individual case basis, with consideration of tendon shape, location, and degree of tissue disruption from the initiating trauma.

Tendon lengthening

In chronic tendon injuries with contracture of the associated muscle, a tendon lengthening procedure may be necessary for apposition without a gap. The Z tenotomy ("sliding Z plasty"), V-Y plasty, and accordion techniques are suggested for gaps greater than 3 cm (Fig. 6) [1,39].

Enhancement of tendon healing

Research revolves around the development of techniques to enhance tendon healing, providing earlier return to more normal function. Several techniques

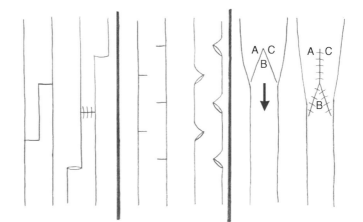

Fig. 6. Tendon lengthening procedures. (*Left to right*) sliding Z plasty, accordion, and V-Y plasty.

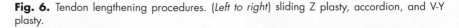

and materials have been reported, including stainless steel tendon anchors for anastomosis [47], bone screws with washers [48], high-density type I collagen bone anchors for reconstruction of bone-tendon interface [49], bioabsorbable interference screws [50], and poly-L-lactic acid bioabsorbable implants [51] for anastomosis and small bone plates [52] sutured across the appositional site to support the anastomosis. Stainless steel tendon anastomosis stabilizing coil anchors (Teno-Fix Tendon Repair System; Ortheon Medical, Winter Park, Florida) are reported in human patients, with the advantage of less adhesion formation [53]. To the author's knowledge, there are no reports of their use in the veterinary literature.

In cases of chronic tendon injury with muscle contracture and gap formation, grafting techniques have been reported to support and enhance healing of the anastomosis site [15]. Donor tissue sources include autologous fascia lata and autologous or allogenous tendon. A canine study [54] reported successful use of a free autologous fascia lata graft for a ruptured CCT in a 3-month-old puppy. An equine study [55] concluded that free autologous sections of tendon placed at a tenotomy site resulted in a sixfold increase in strength between 4 and 8 weeks after surgery. Three bovine studies [56–58] confirmed increased vascularization of the anastomotic site with plasma-preserved tendon allograft.

Injection of substances at the anastomotic site has also been researched. A study in chicken tendon comparing the effects of wrapping amniotic membrane and injecting hyaluronic acid around the anastomotic site found less adhesion formation [59]. Autogenous nonvascularized free flaps of greater omentum augmented angiogenesis and accelerated healing in canine superficial flexor tendon [60]. Injection of platelet concentrate within rat Achilles tendon after transection without surgical repair revealed a 30% increase in tendon callus strength and confirmed greater maturation of the callus histologically [61]. Preliminary testing of injection of urinary bladder matrix powder (Acell-*Vet*, Acell Inc., Jessup, Maryland) suspension within equine suspensory ligament revealed encouraging clinical results [62]. Recombinant equine growth hormone injection intramuscularly had no in vitro effect but did have a negative in vivo effect on biomechanical properties in early phases of tendon healing [63,64]. Intramuscular injection of polysulfated glycosaminoglycans enhanced healing in eight horses with collagenase-induced tendinitis [65].

Modulation of important mediators of wound healing, such as lactate and transforming growth factor-β levels, may reduce adhesion formation in flexor tendon healing [66]. Modulation of the nuclear factor–kappaB gene may increase production of type I collagen, enhancing tensile strength of healing tendon [67]. Cell therapy with bone marrow stromal cells packed into bone tunnels resulted in more perpendicular collagen fiber formation and increased type II collagen at 4 weeks after surgery in rabbits [68]. Engineered tissue replacement has been reported with promising results in vitro in rat Achilles tendon [69]. Many recent advances in tendon injury management may be proven experimentally and become clinically available in the future [70].

Postoperative management

Immobilization of the affected joint is controversial but recommended and is performed in most veterinary case reports for support of tendon anastomosis techniques. A study of Achilles tendon injuries in human patients advocates limited immobilization and early postoperative movement so as to inhibit muscle contracture, increase early tendon strength, and allow early return to function with no increased risk of rupture recurrence [71]. Joint immobilization can be deleterious if prolonged. Immobilization longer than 3 weeks can result in greater articular valgus or varus deformity on discontinuation of joint support [72]. Generally, a 3-week period of complete immobilization is recommended, followed by another 3 weeks of less immobilization to provide a gradual increase in load on the tendon. Some researchers suggest intra-articular hyaluronate injections and supplementation with chondroprotective agents to prevent degenerative articular changes [73]. Immobilization techniques reported include external coaptation with casts or splints, a transarticular screw (calcaneotibial screw), an external fixator boot, transarticular external fixators, and a modified transarticular external fixator. There are advantages and disadvantages of each.

External coaptation can consist of splints, full casts, or cranial or caudal half-casts and primarily applies to CCT injuries. Materials include preformed splints, rolled casts, or thermoplastics. Impaired wound management, increased limb muscle atrophy, and development of pressure sores are the primary disadvantages of external coaptation [39]. The cranial half-cast allows limited movement of the Achilles mechanism, which may reduce complications associated with tarsocrural immobilization. A study of cranial half-casts in five dogs weighing between 20.5 and 35 kg reported that eight layers of cast material were necessary [73]. External fixator boots can cause similar problems as casts [74].

Transarticular screws are surgically placed temporarily between the calcaneus and tibia and should be supported with external coaptation. One study noted an improved outcome compared with casting alone [75]. Removal under general anesthesia is required at the end of the complete immobilization period [39].

Transarticular external fixators consist of two pins placed in the distal tibia and metatarsals for CCT injuries or in the humerus and radius for triceps tendon injuries, resulting in complete hock or elbow joint immobilization. These devices result in greater loss of articular cartilage proteoglycan content compared with casts; therefore, they should only be used for the first 21 days while fibroplasia progresses [76]. A modified transarticular external fixator with pins in the distal tibia and calcaneus has been reported to impede hock flexion successfully while avoiding complications with metatarsal pin placement [77].

POSTOPERATIVE REHABILITATION

The benefits of postoperative rehabilitation in small animal surgery are gradually becoming realized [78]. With respect to biceps tenodesis or CCT injury, patients' postoperative weight bearing and surgeons' immobilization techniques and requested protocols are variable. Therefore, rehabilitation programs must be individually tailored. A suggested protocol for rehabilitation after arthroscopy of the shoulder has been published [79].

Biceps tenodesis patients can present with a "shoulder hike" and resistance to circumduction. The goals of rehabilitation are to strengthen the brachialis muscle as a secondary stabilizer of the joint and to perform gait retraining. CCT healing can be monitored with ultrasound once external coaptation is removed. Low-stress propulsion can generally be performed 8 to 10 weeks after surgery with the goal of realignment of collagen fibers to strengthen the anastomotic site (Caroline P. Adamson, MSPT, CCRP, personal communication, 2004).

SUMMARY

The recognition, diagnosis, and surgical management of tendon conditions, such as bicipital tenosynovitis or CCT injury, have been highlighted in this article. Patient prognosis is variable; however, new research with techniques to provide enhancement of tendon healing may improve outcomes in the near future. Patient rehabilitation is encouraged in all cases for the best results.

References

[1] Harari J. Tendon injuries. In: Surgical complications and wound healing in small animal practice. Philadelphia: WB Saunders; 1993. p. 186–95.

[2] Chaplin DM. The vascular anatomy within normal tendons, divided tendons, free grafts and pedicle tendon grafts in rabbits. J Bone Joint Surg Br 1973;55B:369–89.

[3] Battaglia TC, Clark RT, Chhabra A, et al. Ultrastructural determinants of murine Achilles tendon strength during healing. Connect Tissue Res 2003;44(5):218–24.

[4] Lin TW, Cardenas L, Soslowsky LJ. Biomechanics of tendon injury and repair. J Biomech 2004;37:865–77.

[5] Butler DL, Juncosa N, Dressler MR. Functional efficacy of tendon repair processes. Annu Rev Biomed Eng 2004;6:303–29.

[6] Montgomery RD. Healing of muscle, ligaments and tendons. Semin Vet Med Surg (Small Anim) 1989;4(4):304–11.

[7] Johnston D. Tendons, skeletal muscles, and ligaments in health and disease. In: Newton CP, Nunamaker DM, editors. Textbook of small animal orthopedics. Available at: http://cal. vet.upenn.edu/saortho/chapter04/04mast.htm.

[8] Gelberman RH, Menon J, Gonsalves M, et al. The effects of mobilization on the vascularization of healing flexor tendons in dogs. Clin Orthop 1980;153:283–9.

[9] Mason ML, Allen H. The rate of healing of tendons and experimental study of tensile strength. Ann Surg 1941;113:424–56.

[10] Benjamin M, Hillen B. Mechanical influences on cells, tissues and organs—'mechanical morphogenesis.' Eur J Morphol 2003;41(1):3–7.

[11] Gelberman RH, Vande Berg JS, Lundborg GN, et al. Flexor tendon healing and restoration of gliding surface, and ultrastructure study in dogs. J Bone Joint Surg Am 1980;65A:70–80.

[12] Schulz KS. Forelimb lameness in the adult patient. Vet Clin North Am Small Anim Pract 2001;31(1):85–99.

[13] Cook JL. Forelimb lameness in the young patient. Vet Clin North Am Small Anim Pract 2001;31(1):55–83.

[14] Bardet JF. Diagnosis of shoulder instability in dogs and cats: a retrospective study. J Am Anim Hosp Assoc 1998;34:42–54.

[15] Aron DN. Tendons. In: Bojrab MJ, editor. Current techniques in small animal surgery. Philadelphia: Lea & Febiger; 1990. p. 549–61.

[16] Sidaway BK, McLaughlin RM, Elder SH, et al. The roles of the biceps brachii tendon, the infraspinatus tendon, and the medial glenohumeral ligament as passive stabilizers in the canine shoulder joint. In: Proceedings of the 2004 Conference of the American College of Veterinary Surgeons. Bethesda (MD): American College of Veterinary Surgeons; 2004. p. 20.

[17] Kramer M, Gerwing M, Sheppard C, et al. Ultrasonography for the diagnosis of diseases of the tendon and tendon sheath of the biceps brachii muscle. Vet Surg 2001;30:64–71.

[18] Bardet JF. Lesions of the biceps tendon diagnosis and classification. A retrospective study of 25 cases in 23 dogs and one cat. Vet Comp Orthop Traumatol 1999;12:188–95.

[19] Beale BS, Hulse DA, Schulz KS, et al. Arthroscopically assisted surgery of the shoulder joint. In: Small animal arthroscopy. Philadelphia: WB Saunders; 2003. p. 23–49.

[20] Stobie D, Wallace LJ, Lipowitz AJ, et al. Chronic bicipital tenosynovitis in dogs: 29 cases(1985–1992). J Am Vet Med Assoc 1995;207(2):201–7.

[21] Muir P, Goldsmid SE, Rothwell TLW, et al. Calcifying tendinopathy of the biceps brachii in a dog. J Am Vet Med Assoc 1992;201(11):1747–9.

[22] Rivers B, Wallace L, Johnston GR. Biceps tenosynovitis in the dog: radiographic and sonographic findings. Vet Comp Orthop Traumatol 1992;5:51–7.

[23] Brinker WO, Piermattei DL, Flo GL. Handbook of small animal orthopedics and fracture treatment. 2nd edition. Philadelphia: WB Saunders; 1992. p. 472–96.

[24] Whittick WG. Canine orthopedics. 2nd edition. Philadelphia: WB Saunders; 1990. p. 770–2.

[25] Wall CR, Taylor R. Arthroscopic biceps brachii tenotomy as a treatment for canine bicipital tenosynovitis. J Am Anim Hosp Assoc 2002;38(2):169–75.

[26] Holsworth IG, Schulz KS. Cadaveric evaluation of canine arthroscopic bicipital tenotomy. Vet Comp Orthop Traumatol 2002;15(4):215–22.

[27] Esterline ML, Armbrust LJ, Roush JK. Minimally invasive transection of the canine bicipital tendon. In: Proceedings of the 2004 Conference of the American College of Veterinary Surgeons. Bethesda (MD): American College of Veterinary Surgeons; 2004. p. 7.

[28] Cook JL. Proposed protocol for shoulder assessment in dogs. In: Proceedings of the 2004 Conference of the American College of Veterinary Surgeons. Bethesda (MD): American College of Veterinary Surgeons; 2004. p. 341–3.

[29] Mauterer JV, Prata RG, Carberry CA, et al. Displacement of the tendon of the superficial digital flexor muscle in dogs: 10 cases (1983–1991). J Am Vet Med Assoc 1993; 203(8):1162–5.

[30] Gemmill TJ, Carmichael S. Complete patellar ligament replacement using a fascia lata autograft in a dog. J Small Anim Pract 2003;44(10):456–9.

[31] Smith MEH, de Haan JJ, Peck J, et al. Augmented primary repair of patellar ligament rupture in three dogs. Vet Comp Orthop Traumatol 2000;13(3):154–7.

[32] Meutstege FJ. The classification of canine Achilles' tendon lesions. Vet Comp Orthop Traumatol 1993;6:53–5.

[33] Reinke JD, Mughannam AJ, Owens JM. Avulsion of the gastrocnemius tendon in 11 dogs. J Am Anim Hosp Assoc 1993;29:410–8.

[34] Khan RJ, Fick D, Brammar TJ, et al. Interventions for treating acute Achilles tendon ruptures. Cochrane Database Syst Rev 2004;3:CD003674.

[35] Guerin S, Burbidge H, Firth E, et al. Achilles tenorrhaphy in five dogs: a modified surgical technique and evaluation of a cranial half cast. Vet Comp Orthop Traumatol 1998;11:205–10.

[36] Boothe HW. Suture materials, tissue adhesives, staplers and ligating clips. In: Slatter D, editor. Textbook of small animal surgery. 3rd edition. Philadelphia: WB Saunders; 2003. p. 235–44.

[37] Hatanaka H, Manske PR. Effect of suture size on locking and grasping flexor tendon repair techniques. Clin Orthop 2000;375:267–74.

[38] Berg RJ, Egger E. In vitro comparison of the three loop pulley and locking loop suture patterns for repair of canine weight bearing tendons and collateral ligaments. Vet Surg 1986;15(1):107–10.

[39] Sivacolundhu RK, Marchevsky AM, Read RA, et al. Achilles mechanism reconstruction in 4 dogs. Vet Comp Orthop Traumatol 2001;14:25–31.

[40] Moores AP, Owen MR, Tarlton JF. The three-loop pulley suture versus two locking loop sutures for the repair of canine Achilles tendons. Vet Surg 2004;33:131–7.

[41] Pijanowski GF, Stein LE, Turner TA. Strength characteristics and failure modes of suture patterns in severed goat tendons. Vet Surg 1989;18(5):335–9.

[42] Smith AM, Evans DM. Biomechanical assessment of a new type of flexor tendon repair. J Hand Surg [Am] 2001;26:217–9.

[43] Jassem M, Rose AT, Meister K, et al. Biomechanical analysis of the effect of varying suture pitch in tendon graft fixation. Am J Sports Med 2001;29:734–7.

[44] Renberg WR, Radlinsky MG. In vitro comparison of the locking loop and continuous cruciate suture patterns. Vet Comp Orthop Traumatol 2001;14(1):15–8.

[45] Montgomery RD, Barnes SL, Wenzel JGW, et al. In vitro comparison of the Krackow and locking loop suture patterns for tenorrhaphy of flat tendons. Vet Comp Orthop Traumatol 1994;7:31–4.

[46] Fossum TW. Biomaterials, suturing and hemostasis. In: Small animal surgery. 2nd edition. St. Louis: Mosby; 2002. p. 43–59.

[47] Lewis N, Quitkin HM. Strength analysis and comparison of the Teno Fix tendon repair system with the two-strand modified Kessler repair in the Achilles tendon. Foot Ankle Int 2003;24(11):857–60.

[48] Adamiak Z, Szalecki P. Treatment of bicipital tenosynovitis with double tenodesis. J Small Anim Pract 2003;44(12):539–40.

[49] Walsh WR, Harrison JA, Van Sickle D, et al. Patellar tendon-to-bone healing using high-density collagen bone anchor at 4 years in a sheep model. Am J Sports Med 2004; 32(1):91–5.

[50] Khan W, Agarwal M, Funk L. Repair of distal biceps tendon rupture with a Biotenodesis screw. Arch Orthop Trauma Surg 2004;124(3):206–8.

[51] Eliashar E, Schamme MC, Schumacher J, et al. Use of bioabsorbable implant for repair of severed digital flexor tendons in four horses. Vet Rec 2001;148(16):506–9.

[52] Johnson AL, Hulse D. Management of muscle and tendon injury or disease. In: Fossum TW, editor. Small animal surgery. 2nd edition. St. Louis: Mosby; 2002. p. 1158–67.

[53] Gordon L, Tolar M, Rao KT, et al. Flexor tendon repair using a stainless steel internal anchor. Biomechanical study on human cadaver tendons. J Hand Surg [Am] 1998;23:37–40.

[54] Shani J, Shahar R. Repair of chronic complete traumatic rupture of the common calcaneal tendon in a dog, using a fascia lata graft. Case report and literature review. Vet Comp Orthop Traumatol 2000;13:104–8.

[55] Reiners SR, Jann HW, Stein LE, et al. An evaluation of two autologous tendon grafting techniques in ponies. Vet Surg 2004;31:155–66.

[56] Kumar N, Sharma AK, Sharma AK, et al. Carbon fibres and plasma-preserved tendon allografts for gap repair of flexor tendon in bovines: gross, microscopic and scanning electron microscopic observations. J Vet Med A Physiol Pathol Clin Med 2002;49:269–76.

[57] Kumar N, Sharma AK, Singh GR, et al. Carbon fibres and plasma-preserved tendon allografts for gap repair of flexor tendon in bovines: clinical, radiological and angiographical observations. J Vet Med 2002;49:161–8.

[58] Ramesh R, Kumar N, Sharma AK, et al. Acellular and glutaraldehyde-preserved tendon allografts for reconstruction of superficial digital flexor tendon in bovines: part II—gross, microscopic and scanning electron microscopic observations. J Vet Med A Physiol Pathol Clin Med 2003;50(10):520–6.

[59] Ozgenel GY. The effects of combination of hyaluronic acid and amniotic membrane on the formation of peritendinous adhesions after flexor tendon surgery in chickens. J Bone Joint Surg Br 2004;86(2):301–7.

[60] Oloumi MM, Derakhsahnfar A, Hosseinnia H. The role of autogenous greater omentum in experimental tendon healing in the dog, a histopathologic study. In: Proceedings of the World Small Animal Veterinary Association. World Small Animal Veterinary Association; 2001. p. 44–5.

[61] Aspenberg P, Virchenko O. Platelet concentrate injection improves Achilles tendon repair in rats. Acta Orthop Scand 2004;75(1):93–9.

[62] Mitchell RD. Treatment of tendon and ligament injuries with UBM powder (Acell-Vet®). In: Proceedings of the 2004 Conference of the American College of Veterinary Surgeons. Bethesda (MD): American College of Veterinary Surgeons; 2004. p. 190–3.

[63] Dowling BA, Dart AJ, Hodgson DR, et al. Recombinant equine growth hormone does not affect the in vitro biomechanical properties of equine superficial digital flexor tendon. Vet Surg 2002;31:325–30.

[64] Dowling BA, Dart AJ, Hodgson DR, et al. The effect of recombinant equine growth hormone on the biomechanical properties of healing superficial digital flexor tendons in horses. Vet Surg 2002;31:320–4.

[65] Redding WR, Booth LC, Pool RR. The effects of polysulphated glycosaminoglycan on the healing of collagenase induced tendinitis. Vet Comp Orthop Traumatol 1999;12:48–55.

[66] Yalamanchi N, Klein MB, Pham HM, et al. Flexor tendon wound healing in vitro: lactate up-regulation of TGF-beta expression and functional activity. Plast Reconstr Surg 2004;113(2):625–32.

[67] Tang JB, Xu Y, Ding F, et al. Expression of genes for collagen production and NF-kappaB gene activation of in vivo healing flexor tendons. J Hand Surg [Am] 2004;29(4):564–70.

[68] Ouyang HW, Goh JC, Lee EH. Use of bone marrow stromal cells for tendon graft-to-bone healing: histological and immunohistochemical studies in a rabbit model. Am J Sports Med 2004;32(2):321–7.

[69] Calve S, Dennis RG, Kosnik PE, et al. Engineering of functional tendon. Tissue Eng 2004;10(5/6):755–61.

[70] Dahlgren LA. Recent advances in the treatment of tendon injuries. In: Proceedings of the 2004 Conference of the American College of Veterinary Surgeons. Bethesda (MD): American College of Veterinary Surgeons; 2004. p. 316–20.

[71] Mandelbaum BR, Myerson MS, Forster R. Achilles tendon ruptures. A new method of repair, early range of motion and functional rehabilitation. Am J Sports Med 1995;23:392–5.

[72] Montgomery R, Fitch R. Muscle and tendon disorders. In: Slatter D, editor. Textbook of small animal surgery. 3rd edition. Philadelphia: WB Saunders; 2003. p. 2264–72.

[73] Hulse DA, Aron DN. Advances in small animal orthopedics. Compend Contin Educ Pract Vet 1994;16(7):831–2.

[74] Gallagher LA, Rudy RL, Smeak DD. The external fixator boot: application principles, techniques, and indications. J Am Anim Hosp Assoc 1990;26:403–9.

[75] Worth AJ, Danielsson F, Bray JP, et al. Common calcanean tendon injuries in working dogs in New Zealand. N Z Vet J 2004;52(3):109–16.

[76] Behrens F, Kraft EL, Oegema TR. Biochemical changes in articular cartilage after joint immobilization by casting or external fixation. J Orthop Res 1989;7:335–43.

[77] de Haan JJ, Goring RL, Renberg C, et al. Modified transarticular external skeletal fixation for support of Achilles tenorrhaphy in four dogs. Vet Comp Orthop Traumatol 1995;8:32–5.

[78] Marsolais GS, Dvorak G, Conzemius MG. Effects of postoperative rehabilitation on limb function after cranial cruciate ligament repair in dogs. J Am Vet Med Assoc 2002; 220(9):1325–30.

[79] Arthroscopically assisted surgery of the shoulder joint. In: Beale B, Hulse DA, Schulz KS, et al, editors. Small animal arthroscopy. Philadelphia: WB Saunders; 2003. p. 26.

Vet Clin Small Anim 35 (2005) 1213–1231

VETERINARY CLINICS

SMALL ANIMAL PRACTICE

ELSEVIER
SAUNDERS

Total Joint Replacement in the Dog

Michael G. Conzemius, DVM, PhD*,
Jennifer Vandervoort, DVM

Department of Small Animal Surgery, College of Veterinary Medicine,
Iowa State University, South 16th Street, Ames, IA 50010, USA

HISTORY

The reported use of the cemented total hip replacement (THR) implants in humans began in 1961 [1] and coined Charnley as the "father of modern total hip replacements" [1–4]. Since this initial report, THRs have been performed frequently in human and veterinary patients. A successful report of a fixed-head THR prosthesis (Richard's Canine II Hip Prosthesis, Richards Medical, Memphis, Tennessee) implantation in the dog by Hoefle established THR as a potential treatment option for veterinary patients [5]. Numerous reports followed that documented the use of the fixed-head THR system in the dog with subjectively defined good to excellent results [6–12]. In June 1990, the cemented modular total hip prosthesis (Canine Modular Hip System, Biomedtrix, Boonton, New Jersey) and instrumentation system were introduced. The inception of the modular system improved the surgical technique and provided good clinical results [8,13]. Volumes of clinical and experimental information have accumulated to address implant characteristics and prevention of complications in an effort to improve outcomes further. Recent additions to the veterinary market include other modular cemented systems, but much attention has focused on cementless systems, such as the PCA Canine Total Hip System (Biomedtrix,) and the KYON total hip replacement system (Kyon, Zurich, Switzerland).

INDICATIONS

The primary indication for THR is severe osteoarthritis (OA) in the hip that causes lameness, pain, diminished limb function, and a decrease in the patient's quality of life. It is important to note that severe radiographic disease alone is not an indication for THR. It has been reported that the relationship between radiographic and clinical disease is poor and unpredictable [14]. Although

*Corresponding author. Department of Veterinary Clinical Sciences, College of Veterinary Medicine Iowa State University, South 16th Street, Ames, IA 50010. E-mail address: conz@iastate.edu (M.G. Conzemius).

0195-5616/05/$ – see front matter
doi:10.1016/j.cvsm.2005.05.006

coxofemoral pain is most commonly associated with canine hip dysplasia, it also can be from primary OA unrelated to canine hip dysplasia, chronic hip luxations, failed femoral head and neck ostectomies, severe femoral head or neck fractures, malunions after acetabular, femoral head, or neck fractures, and from avascular necrosis of the femoral head [8]. Although THR can be performed in a wide variety of canine patients, the ideal patient is at least a middle aged, medium or large breed that behaves well enough that it will not reduce the chance of success after surgery. Good client communication before surgery is of paramount importance. Clients must understand the probability for success and failure, understand potential long-term constraints on the patient's activity after surgery, have the ability to follow instructions for postoperative care of the patient, and have the financial resources to pay for what is generally a comparably expensive initial procedure that may have complications that require expensive subsequent procedures. Finally, the surgeon and surgical assistants should be trained adequately in performing THR and be dedicated to all surgical principles (especially asepsis) necessary to optimize the chance for surgical success.

CONTRAINDICATIONS

Perhaps the most commonly encountered contraindication for THR is concurrent orthopedic disease in the affected limb. Frequently, patients present with a history of unilateral rear limb lameness, and radiographs document the presence of severe hip OA. When a patient presents for THR, the physical examination should be used to confirm that presence of hip pain and the absence of stifle pain. Clinicians should be especially careful when the patient history and physical examination include documentation of unilateral rear limb lameness. When a patient has pain from a torn cranial cruciate ligament and hip OA, performing THR alone rarely improves the patient's limb function. In general, I perform surgery to address the stifle pain first.

Neurologic dysfunction in the proposed THR limb is a contraindication if the neurologic disease is progressive or will affect outcome. A German Shepherd dog with degenerative myelopathy and severe hip OA is a good example of a patient that should not undergo THR. Similarly, a dog with clinical signs associated with lumbosacral disease should not undergo THR until after the lumbosacral problems are resolved.

Ongoing local or systemic infection increases the probability of operative contamination and bacteremia, which are contraindications to THR. Pyoderma that is in the operative field should be treated and resolved before surgery. Likewise, the patient should be evaluated for clinical signs of bacterial cystitis, gingivitis, and otitis externa before surgery. Previous surgery at the hip is not necessarily a contraindication, but the owners should be informed that prior joint surgeries likely will double the chance for infection [15]. Previous surgeries may complicate the surgical procedure by changing anatomic landmarks and increasing periarticular fibrosis. THR can be performed successfully after triple pelvic osteotomy or femoral head and neck excision, although it is not encouraged because these procedures may have higher complication rates.

Total joint replacement historically has not been performed in veterinary patients that have neoplasia. This practice, however, has changed as patient owners and veterinary oncology have evolved. Although we are not aware of any publications that address allograft prosthetic composites in veterinary patients, they are commonly performed in human medicine and provide another treatment option in patients with joint tumors [16]. We suggest that other variables that increase the probability for failure include the patient not being skeletally mature and the patient or owners not being able to restrict the dog's activity after surgery.

CEMENTED HIP REPLACEMENT SYSTEMS

Historically, THR systems that require cement fixation of the implants have been the most popular in veterinary practice. Although several systems are commercially available, the design modifications among the group are small but arguably important. Common implant features to which surgeons must pay close attention include materials used (each component and cement), manufacturing and processing practices of the company, and history of the implant design. These features are detailed in this section, but many of the concepts can be applied to all THR systems.

In the veterinary field, femoral components can be made from stainless steel, cobalt-chromium, or titanium. Each alloy has particular mechanical, metallurgic, and immunogenic advantages and disadvantages because they have excellent mechanical properties, are resistant to corrosion, and are relatively inert in the body. Immune hypersensitivity to metal implants (eg, nickel and chromium) has been reported in people, but more recent evidence suggests that this occurs in only a small percentage of patients and has no impact on the rate of aseptic loosening [17,18]. Titanium femoral components, which have a comparably smaller modulus of elasticity, were used for a short period of time in veterinary medicine, but when cemented they have been shown to be loosely associated with an increased rate of aseptic loosening in the dog [19].

The shape of the femoral stem also can impact outcome, and there are significant variations among the commercially available systems [20]. Increasing the length of the femoral stem increases the probability that the stem tip will be in contact with the distal femoral cortex [21]. It is undesirable to have the implant in direct contact with the bone because it has been correlated with an increased rate of aseptic loosening in the dog and it decreases the size of the cement mantle [19]. Mechanically, the larger the cement mantle the better, because increased cement mantle thickness around the femoral stem increases the fatigue life of a bone implant system by reducing peak strains within the cement [22]. The simple decision to use a short femoral stem also can be incorrect, however, because although a shorter implant has a potential to improve implant fit, it leads to significantly higher cement strains that may increase the risk for aseptic loosening [23]. Proximal to distal curvature to improve implant fit in the curved canine femur is a feature of some implant systems and improves the probability that the implant will be cemented in a centralized position [20]. The decision regarding what stem length to use in an individual patient must be balanced, and we suggest that surgeons use the longest femoral implant that stills allow for centralization of the implant and a cement mantle thickness of at least 2 mm. Implant centralization also can be achieved using a centralizer, which is commercially available with some systems or can be achieved at the time of surgery using extra cement.

Other significant design variations that have been investigated and create some controversy are proximal implant collars, flanges, and stem surface roughness. To the best of the authors' knowledge, all of the veterinary cemented designs have a collared femoral component that rests on the proximal-medial aspect of the femoral osteotomy site. The collar's role is to assist in implant positioning and increase bone implant surface area and proportionally reduce stress in an effort to reduce the incidence and severity of component subsidence if implant loosening occurs. Proximal femoral implant flanges have been shown to increase the interlock between the stem and the cement and decrease the proximal-medial stress shielding [24]. This advantage comes at a cost, however. The motion per cycle of flanged stems within a cement mantle is smaller than that of nonflanged stems; however, the motion per cycle of the cement mantle within the femoral canal is greater with the flanged stems than with the nonflanged stems [24]. This puts the cement mantle at risk and may be detrimental to the survival of the implant. Surface roughness of the femoral component is important because retrieval studies suggest that the loosening process of the cemented femoral components of total hip arthroplasties is initiated by failure of the bond between the prosthesis and the cement mantle [25]. High interface friction at the stem-cement interface, which to some degree corresponds to a degree of surface roughness, has the capacity to reduce debonding stresses. Debonded rough stems produce more cement damage than polished ones, however, and some literature suggests that polished stems are clinically superior with respect to stems with a mat surface finish [25]. Many of the veterinary THR systems have straight femoral stems tapered only in the coronal plane. Given this implant design, it has been demonstrated that a rough surface offers the advantage of less per-cycle motion and a decreased rate of migration over the course of cyclic loading [26]. Although this topic always will be somewhat controversial, some researchers suggest that stems should have either a polished microstructure to minimize the local cement stresses or a significant macrostructure to minimize micromotion at the stem-cement interface [25].

The femoral head is the second component used on the femoral side. Although some systems use a single implant on the femoral side that has the head attached to the femoral stem, most have the femoral head as a separate implant. When separate, the femoral head is generally attached to the stem by a simple taper fit in which the neck of the femoral stem has a wider taper angle than the female, taper hole on the nonarticular portion of the femoral head component. The primary advantage of separate femoral components is that it allows for a modular system. In effect, the femoral head can have receptive holes with varying taper angles on the femoral neck. (The femoral-neck-to-femoral-shaft angle remains the same. What changes is the taper portion of the femoral neck.) This design allows for the surgeon to shorten or lengthen the functional neck length of the system. This option is useful at the time of surgery. The disadvantage is that it creates a metal-on-metal articulation that has some micromotion and corrosion and creates particulate wear debris. Surgeons also should be aware of the finishing polish on the femoral head and confirm with the manufacturer that the implants conform to the standards of the American Society for Testing and Materials.

The acetabular cup is composed of ultrahigh molecular weight polyethylene and should be machined with an articular surface that abides by American Society for Testing and Materials standards. To the best of the authors' knowledge, all of the veterinary cemented systems use a single implant system on the acetabular side, which simplifies surgical technique and avoids the formation of secondary wear debris between a ultra-high molecular weight polyethylene (UHMWPE) cup and a metal backing implant. The articular size of the cup can vary but must balance the fact that metal-UHMWPE articulations that are too small increase the probability of luxation and that as the articulation increases in size, the surface area of the articulation increases, which increases the amount of wear debris and frequency of aseptic loosening [27]. Puolakka and colleagues [28] reported that a simple increase in acetabular cup size from 28 mm to 32 mm doubled the rate of volumetric wear. The significance of wear rates are that for every 0.1 mm/y increase in the linear wear rate, the likelihood of the development of osteolysis increases by a factor of four [27]. Although this factor is critical for people who receive THR, the significance of this for veterinary patients is still unknown. Skurla and James [13] compared acetabular wear rates in dogs to humans and reported that cup wear rates were reduced by nearly 50% in dogs. This fact should not be surprising because acetabular cup sizes are proportionally smaller and veterinary patients are quadrupeds, which reduces surface area and mechanical load, respectively. Acetabular cup design can impact the frequency of dislocation, however, which is generally associated with surgical technique or postoperative trauma and is addressed in the section on complications.

The final implant is, in the authors' opinion, the weakest link in cemented implant systems. In veterinary medicine, the cement mantle is generally made from polymethylmethacrylate (PMMA), which is biomechanically weaker than the other implants used in the system. This originates from the fact that PMMA is comparatively weak in bending, the cement mantle is not nearly as thick as other implants used, it sees proportionally high bending stresses, and it is in direct contact with bone, which has the capacity to remodel from what was once in direct contact with bone and is stable to PMMA that is in contact with fibrous tissue and unstable. These factors predispose the cement mantle to early failure and aseptic loosening, which suggests that selection of cement and cementing technique perhaps play a greater role in outcome than implant design.

Several factors are important for a successful cement mantle. First, one should select PMMA that has a polymeric exothermic reaction that liberates heat below the temperature that causes osteocyte death and bone remodeling. The critical thermal factors for bone necrosis depend on temperature and duration of exposure. It takes approximately 380 seconds for a temperature of 50°C or 60 seconds for a temperature of 70°C to kill osteocytes [29]. Thermal necrosis of bone can be managed, in part, by controlling the thickness of the cement mantle. The temperature profiles in the bone cement prosthesis system have shown that the thicker the cement, the higher the peak temperature in the bone. In one report, cement mantle that reached 7 mm thick had a predicted peak temperature of more than 55°C [30]. This information should be used with caution; cement mantle thickness increases in bending strength to the third power each time it doubles in thickness. Another technique for reducing thermal heating is water cooling. In one publication, continuous irrigation with Ringer's solution reduced mean temperature by 9°C when compared with no irrigation [31].

Second, one should select PMMA that allows for cementing during the liquid phase. Cement penetration into the small pores of cortical and cancellous bone strongly influence interface strength, and it has been reported that as cement viscosity decreases, bone cement push-out strength increases [32]. In practice, most of the commercially available brands have a liquid phase that is functionally long enough to insert in a liquid phase. Surgeons who elect to implant cement in the dough (high-viscosity) phase reduce the strength of the cement-bone interface, however, and likely risk an increase in the rate of aseptic loosening. The cement-bone interface also can be improved by injecting the cement under pressure, although in practice this can be achieved only in the femur. The easiest way to create pressure is with the use of a cement restrictor to occlude the intramedullary canal. Cement restrictors occlude the femoral canal, increase intramedullary pressures, and increase cement stability and reduce cement leakage [33].

Third, one should use cement preparation techniques that minimize air bubbles and cracks in the cement mantle. Strong evidence exists that cracks in the cement are initiated at voids that act as stress risers, particularly at the cement-stem interface [34,35]. The preferential formation of voids at this site results from shrinkage during polymerization and the initiation of this process at the warmer cement-bone interface, which causes bone cement to shrink away from the stem [34]. This process creates debonding of the cement from metal implants and has been implicated in the loosening of cemented total hip prostheses [34]. Debonding can be reduced by preheating the femoral stem. Stems preheated to a minimum of 37°C have greater interface shear strength than stems inserted at room temperature initially (53% greater strength) and after simulated aging (155% greater strength) [29]. Fatigue lifetimes are also improved, and there is a more than 99% decrease in cement-stem interface porosity. The setting time of the cement decreased 12% and the maximum temperature at the cement-bone interface increased 6°C. Polymerization temperatures at the cement-bone interface also increased [29]. Although there is a risk that the increase in temperature of the bone will create more osteocyte death, at least in one report this was not the case [34]. There is no benefit to prewarming acetabular cups before implantation [36].

Fourth, one should minimize additives to the PMMA when appropriate. Barium sulfate is added to PMMA as a radiopacifier. It has been reported that barium sulfate additions reduce the fatigue strength of PMMA when compared with plain PMMA [37]. One report that investigated the in vitro effects of barium sulfate on cells also suggested that barium sulfate damaged cultured cells at a 1-hour endpoint [38]. Antibiotics, such as gentamicin, are added to bone cement to treat or prevent infection in arthroplasty. Whereas some researchers report that the addition of gentamicin sulfate has no detrimental effect to PMMA [37], others suggest that the addition of antibiotics reduces the compression strength of PMMA [39,40]. It is important to note that in general, PMMA/antibiotic composites inhibit bacterial growth of susceptible bacteria for 7 to 10 days [40].

The final consideration, although there are arguably others, is vacuum preparation of the cement. During cement preparation, all staff in the operating theater are exposed to PMMA fumes, which are known to have toxic side effects [41]. Vacuum mixing of bone cement significantly reduces the emission of MMA vapors in the breathing zone when compared with classic hand mixing in an open bowl [41]. Vacuum preparation of cement also has been reported to provide consistent porosity reduction in cement mantle [42]. One should recognize, however, that there is debate in the literature because it also has been reported that vacuum mixing does not seem to reduce cement prosthesis interface porosity or improve its mechanical properties [43].

NONCEMENTED HIP REPLACEMENT SYSTEMS

Two mechanisms to achieve cementless THR are popular in veterinary medicine. The first mechanism achieves short-term stability via press-fit of the components into the prepared bone and long-term stability by porous ingrowth of new bone into a metal, porous surface on the components surfaces. Noncemented, or cementless, systems are widely used in human orthopedics and have had periodic use in veterinary surgery for more than 20 years. Because bone cement is not used as a stabilizer, preparation of the bone beds of the femur and acetabulum are critical and, in the authors' opinion, increase the level of technical difficulty for the surgeon. This process requires identifying anatomic landmarks and reproducibly creating bone beds that are capable of receiving a press-fit implant. If the components are positioned in an anatomic position and have sufficient stability in their bone beds, limb function will be adequate and new bone will grow into their osteoconductive surfaces and create an excellent—and arguably superior—biologic prosthetic system [44–46]. DeYoung and colleagues [44] used a porous-coated modular total hip system in

92 patients and reported that a short-term successful outcome was achieved 98% of the time. This high rate of success is encouraging, but one must remember that follow-up time was limited to only 3 months after surgery. They stated that problems can occur and that this type of component is not ideal for all patients [44].

Subsequently, a long-term prospective evaluation of 50 consecutive THR in 41 patients using the same cementless system was performed in which long-term follow-up was available for 37 dogs [47]. In that study, THR survival analysis determined that the 6-year survival rate for the system was 87% and limb function was normal for most successful cases. When gait was abnormal, it was attributed to THR dislocation ($n = 3$), lumbosacral disease ($n = 2$), degenerative myelopathy ($n = 1$), autoimmune disease ($n = 1$), brain tumor ($n = 1$), and osteosarcoma of the femur ($n = 1$) [47]. One interesting finding was that no cases of aseptic loosening were found. This type of prosthetic system is arguably better for some patients. Biologic fixation certainly makes good sense in younger, more active patients that have a greater potential to provide long-term wear and tear on their cement mantles. In contrast, it might be unwise to use porous ingrowth systems in patients that have questionable bone stock, decreased bone mineral mass, or anatomic features that reduce canal fill of the press-fit implant. Femoral morphology that might create a reduced canal fill is likely the most common concern to surgeons who use porous ingrowth systems because the percentage of canal fill is an accurate predictor of component subsidence [48]. Components implanted into femora with a stovepipe morphology (canal flare index ≤ 1.8) were six times more likely to subside than implants in femora that had a normal appearance (canal flare index 1.8–2.5) and 72 times more likely to subside than implants in champagne-fluted femora (canal flare index ≥ 2.5) [48]. This type of femoral anatomy is common in German Shepherd dogs.

An alternative method to achieve short-term stability of the femoral component is via a mechanical interlock system and long-term stability via bone ingrowth. A comparatively new system in veterinary medicine uses a unique interlock system for the femoral component that takes advantage of previously described orthopedic technologies, locking bone plate systems, and interlocking nails. More specifically, monocortical screws lock the femoral stem to the medial cortex of the femur. The proposed advantages of this concept, when compared with press-fit systems, are the initial mechanical strength of the femoral component and the fact that by design one femoral stem size can fit a wide range of patient femur sizes. (One could argue, however, that these are also features of cemented implant systems.) This system also takes advantages of the widely accepted concept that the medial cortex of the femur is the primary load-bearing cortex during weight bearing. The monocortical design of the stem attempts to address the problem of micromotion at the stem-bone interface that occurs as a result of differing mechanical stresses present on the medial versus lateral bone surfaces. This is one mechanism in which aseptic loosening of the femoral component might occur. The acetabular component is a two-piece press-fit component. The acetabular cup design also attempts to address the problem of interface micromotion with a cancellous bone bed by using a comparatively compliant titanium shell. The surface of the titanium shell that opposes bone has holes that permit bone ingrowth for long-term stability.

One controversial design feature of some acetabular components is a polyethylene cup that inserts within the metal shell and leaves a hydraulically open space between the shell and insert. Although it has been suggested that this design allows the convective mechanisms of fluid mass transport to permit bone ingrowth and that this remodeling can only occur if a potential space exists between the shell and the polyethylene liner, much scientific literature would disagree. In one study, Walter and colleagues [49] reported on the pumping of fluid in cementless cups with holes and concluded that cyclic forces, such as those that occur in normal gait, can act on the polyethylene liner, the metal shell, and the supporting bone to pump fluid to create a retroacetabular osteolytic lesion. This pumping action may contribute to the pathogenesis of osteolysis by the mechanisms of fluid pressure, fluid flow, or the transportation of wear particles [49]. Similarly, Manley and colleagues [50] performed a 10-year follow-up on patients that underwent THR that had various acetabular component designs, including that of the design feature in question, and found that pressure fluctuations that occur at the hip or modular components that pump fluid during loading create cyclic pressure changes that may be a causative factor in bone resorption and an increased rate of aseptic loosening. To date, little veterinary literature addresses short- or long-term prognosis using this type of THR design (femoral and acetabular designs).

PERIOPERATIVE CARE

Undoubtedly, one important aspect of surgical technique is strict surgical asepsis. Preoperative care might include checking the patient for systemic infection (eg, otitis externa, cystitis) and local pyoderma. A complete blood count, inspection of the ears and skin, and culture of the urine are commonly recommended. Perioperative antibiotics are required, and a broad-spectrum bactericidal antibiotic should be used. Intraoperative considerations include limiting contamination of the surgical field by covering the limb with an antimicrobial wrap, controlling operative room temperature to limit sweating of the surgeons, using antibiotic-impregnated PMMA, and changing gloves after draping the patient [51,52]. Microbiologic culture of the surgical field is also commonly performed, although some reports suggest that intraoperative cultures correlate poorly with the probability of the patient developing a postoperative complication [53]. In contrast, a positive culture result obtained after opening and when closing the incision is a significant predictor of subsequent infection [54]. After THR we recommend 8 weeks of exercise restriction to limit the probability of seroma formation and hip luxation. Follow-up radiographs after this 8-week time period to identify typical remodeling changes of the bone should direct the future patient's activity level.

COMPLICATIONS

Although most clinical patients achieve good to excellent results after total hip arthroplasty, numerous complications are possible, including luxation, aseptic loosening, infection, and femoral fracture [9,11,55,56]. With improved surgical techniques and experience, the overall complication rate has declined since the inception of total hip arthroplasty in the dog. It is currently estimated that between 3.8% and 11% of all total hip prostheses will develop a complication [9,10,55,56].

Luxations are considered one of the more common complications, and they reportedly occur in 1% to 7% of all total hips that are implanted [12,55,56]. The cause of luxation can originate from surgical error, inappropriate postoperative management, and trauma. Surgical errors include improper positioning of the acetabular or femoral components or the presence of excessive quantities of PMMA that physically do not permit joint congruency [55,57]. Uncontrolled, premature activity in the early (4- to 8-week) postoperative period also can lead to luxation [11,57]. In dogs, luxations occur in the early postoperative period (excluding traumatic luxations), with reports indicating that 63% to 75% of luxations occur within 4 weeks of surgery [7,12]. Treatment for the luxation usually begins with attempts of closed reduction; however, open reduction or repositioning of the prosthesis is generally required.

Infection of a total hip prosthesis usually results in a catastrophic outcome (ie, explantation). Eradication of the infection requires excision of all infected or necrotic tissues and all implants, including cement [58,59]. The incidence of deep infections gradually has declined over the years and is currently estimated to be between 1% and 4.7% [12,56]. Infection after THR can occur secondary to intraoperative contamination, hematogenous infection, or local extension from an infected wound. Clinical variables that increase the probability of infection include increased surgical time (>90 minutes) and increased number of previous surgeries [15,54]. Hematogenous infections uncommonly occur but present a lifelong risk for infection of prosthetics. Dental disease, wound abscesses, pyoderma, urinary tract infection, and discospondylitis are potential sources of hematogenous bacteria.

Aseptic loosening is a major cause of implant failure in human and canine patients with cemented or cementless total joint systems. In humans, 10% to 15% of all THRs require a revision surgery for failed arthroplasties secondary to aseptic loosening [60,61]. The acetabular and femoral components can be affected by this late-term complication. The hallmark of aseptic loosening includes the formation of a synovial-like membrane at the bone-cement interface (for cemented systems) or implant-bone interface (porous ingrowth systems) that histologically appears as a granulomatous foreign body reaction (Fig. 1A, B) [11,61]. In cemented systems, debonding of the components from the bone cement also can occur (Fig. 2). The cause of aseptic loosening is not precisely known; however, multiple mechanisms are associated with it. Implant design, implant position, cementing technique, patient activity level, implant stability, and osseous changes caused by wear particle formation have been

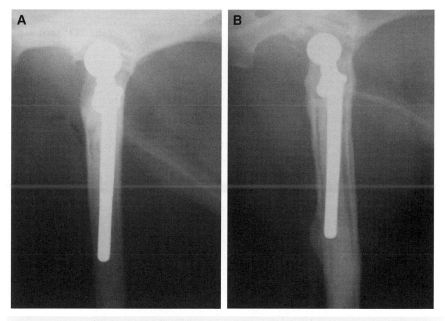

Fig. 1. (A) Lateral radiograph of a THR 8 weeks after surgery. (B) Lateral radiograph (same as Fig. 1A) of a THR 26 months after surgery. Notice the radiolucency at the cement-bone interface and the periosteal reaction at the tip of the femoral stem. Aseptic loosening was diagnosed radiographically.

implicated as playing a role in aseptic loosening [62,63]. A diagnosis of aseptic loosening can be made by physical examination and radiographs. Animals may have varying degrees of lameness, painful coxofemoral range of motion, and pain with palpation of the femoral shaft. The most important radiographic feature of aseptic loosening is an actively widening radiolucent line between the bone and cement or the bone and implant. Other radiographic features of loosening include migration of the femoral stem and axial deviation [61,63].

Femoral fractures can develop intra- or postoperatively. During reaming or broaching of the femoral canal, complete or fissure fractures can be created [11,44]. Fractures most commonly occur (87%) at the end of the rigid implant system because of an elastic modulus mismatch between the implant system and the remaining bone (Fig. 3A–C) [64]. Formation of fissure fractures during the cementless arthroplasty system most commonly occurs during broaching or seating of the femoral stem at the femoral calcar or at intertrochanteric areas [65]. Normally, biomechanical forces are distributed and shared over the entire length of bone after THR forces are more concentrated at the distal aspect of the femoral stem. Over time, remodeling of the femoral diaphysis occurs because of the increased load and the probability of fracture decreases. In people who have undergone THR, the incidence of implant-related fracture is between 1.5% and 3.5% [66–69]. A recent retrospective veterinary study

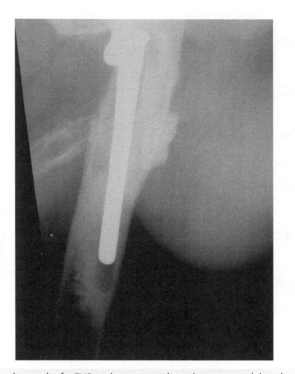

Fig. 2. Lateral radiograph of a THR replacement with implant-cement debonding 4 years after surgery.

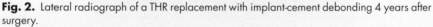

reported a 2.34% (16/684) incidence of femoral fractures after primary THR [64]. It was reported that dogs that developed femoral fractures were generally older (7.4 years) at the time of THR than those without fracture (4.9 years) and that most (57%) of the dogs had bilateral THR. Radiographically apparent fissures caused by femoral reaming or implantation were seen postoperatively in 45% (9/20) of the femurs that developed fractures subsequently.

Predisposing factors for femoral fracture formation include cortical bone thinning caused by osteopathies, aseptic loosening, and previous surgeries [70]. To maintain a low incidence of femoral fractures, a surgeon should select cases carefully, avoid creating fissures, stabilize fissures when recognized (cerclage wires), restrict activity and high-impact exercises, and perform annual re-evaluations of cases so early detection of aseptic loosening and revision surgery can be considered.

Migration of a cementless femoral stem distally within the femoral canal is termed subsidence [48,71]. The severity of subsidence that occurs is related to implant size, stability, friction, and distribution of the implant-bone interface [48,71,72]. Normally 1 to 2 mm of subsidence is expected in the initial postoperative period [71]. Subsidence can be determined by comparison of postoperative and follow-up radiographs. When placing a cementless total hip

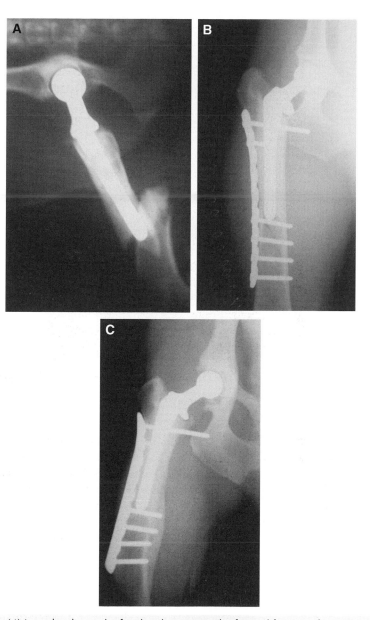

Fig. 3. (*A*) Lateral radiograph of a dog that sustained a femoral fracture after THR near the distal end of the femoral implant and the cement mantle. (*B*) Lateral radiograph of a dog (same as Fig. 3A) immediately after surgery for repair of a femoral fracture. (*C*) Lateral radiograph of a dog (same as Fig. 3A) 1 year after surgery for repair of a femoral fracture.

prosthesis, preoperative planning and templating are crucial to maximize femoral filling and decrease subsidence [47,48,71].

A significant increase in intramedullary pressure occurs during insertion of bone cement into the medullary canal of femur. This increase in pressure has been reported to be as high as 900 mm Hg and can lead to the appearance of medullary contents in the pulmonary system [73–75]. Embolization of bone marrow and fat is believed to be a primary cause of intraoperative complications in humans and results in death. The incidence of symptomatic embolism without death in humans has been reported to be 0.5% [76]. Pulmonary embolism has not been recognized as a common clinical complication in canine patients undergoing implantation of cemented total hips. Few reports of mortality associated with pulmonary fat emboli exist, however [75,76]. Evidence indicates that pulmonary microembolism by medullary contents occurs in large numbers of canine patients during femoral stem insertion. This fact is concluded based on changes in pulmonary function by a decreased end tidal PCO_2 and increased $P(a-ET)CO_2$, embolemia visualized by ultrasonography, and perfusion defects on pulmonary scintigraphy [74,76]. As the numbers of total hip arthroplasties increase in canine patients, the incidence of recognizable pulmonary embolism may be more pronounced.

Reported intrapelvic complications are rare in humans and dogs but include obturator neuropathy, sciatic neuropathy, fistula formation, false aneurysm, hemorrhage/hematoma, and intrapelvic mass formation [77]. False aneurysms or hemorrhages are associated with trauma to the pelvic vasculature, particularly the external iliac artery [77]. Extrusion of large volumes of PMMA through a perforated medial acetabular wall usually results in neuropathies or mass effect. In humans, intrapelvic mass formation is the least common of all intrapelvic THR complications and accounts for 6% (3/50) of the intrapelvic complications. The time from THR to diagnosis of the intrapelvic mass typically lasts years [77]. Sciatic neurapraxia can occur from excessive retraction of the nerve, contact between PMMA and the nerve, or compression caused by hematoma formation. The surgical approach used in the canine patient makes traction on nerve an unlikely occurrence. The exothermic reaction of the cement has been suspected to have resulted in neurapraxia in few canine patients, however. The development of neoplasia has been reported in association with total hip arthroplasty [78,79]. It is possible that the development of osteosarcoma was associated with bone infarction or loose implants in two of the three reports [78,80]. Sarcomas associated with fracture and medullary infarction have been reported before [81–83], although spontaneous neoplasia is most common. A retrospective study reported a 14% incidence (15/110 cases) of femora having radiographic evidence of intramedullary infarction after prosthetic implantation [84]. The incidence of infarction was the same for cemented and uncemented implants. Femoral infarction most likely results from iatrogenic trauma during femoral preparation and stem placement because some lesions developed distal to the implants after surgery.

ATYPICAL TOTAL HIP REPLACEMENT CASES

Although most veterinary patients that undergo THR are medium- to large-breed dogs, occasionally a smaller dog presents and the owners elect THR. The use of a mini-prosthetic system is commercially available and has been reported as being effective [85]. Some patients have pelvic anatomy that requires acetabular augmentation for optimum acetabular cup implantation. When this situation arises, it has been reported that the excised femoral head and neck or the ipsilateral ilial wing can be used as a corticocancellous bone graft to increase the volume of bone available for component implantation [86]. In one report, nine out of ten hips that used this technique had a successful outcome with minimal radiographic and no functional abnormalities [86].

ELBOW REPLACEMENT

Total elbow replacement long has been needed for dogs that suffer from OA of the elbow. To the best of the authors' knowledge, the first peer-reviewed reference that described this technique used a nonconstrained, two-component, cemented system in six research dogs [87]. Although complications occurred in three of six dogs, the remaining three had an excellent outcome and their limb function returned to that of the opposite, unoperated limb. The conclusions from this report were that design and surgical technique must be improved, but total elbow replacement should be considered as a treatment option for dogs

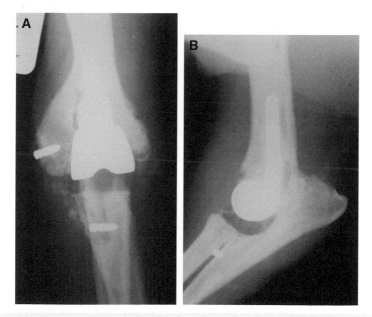

Fig. 4. (A) Craniocaudal radiograph of a dog 12 weeks after having total elbow replacement. (B) Lateral radiograph of a dog (same as Fig. 4A) 12 weeks after total elbow replacement.

with elbow OA and pain. This report was followed by a clinical report using a similar but improved system. In a prospective study of their first 20 patients with severe elbow OA and pain, elbow replacement was successful in 80% of patients 1 year after surgery (Fig. 4A, B) [88]. Complications included infection, fracture, and luxation. After continued improvement in component design, surgical technique, and cutting guides, an improved prognosis has been seen by the authors.

Although many of the general principals of joint replacement (eg, contra-indications, cementing) described for THR apply to elbow replacement, there are some differences. Patient selection should be restricted to include dogs that have a reduced quality of life (eg, joint pain, difficulty walking) on a day-to-day basis even when treated with anti-inflammatory medication. OA in the elbow should be severe. Postoperative care is also a bit different, with postoperative rehabilitation playing a more important role. In the authors' experience, most patients with severe elbow OA have a significantly reduced range of motion in flexion. Although some of this problem can be corrected during surgery; if range of motion is not preserved early in the postoperative period the periarticular fibrosis rapidly returns.

References

[1] Charnley J. Arthroplasty of the hip: a new operation. Lancet 1961;1:1129–32.

[2] Charnley J. Total hip replacement. JAMA 1974;230:1025–8.

[3] Coventry MB, Beckenbaugh RD, Nolan DR, et al. 2,012 total hip arthroplasties: a study of postoperative course and early complications. J Bone Joint Dis 1974;56A:273–84.

[4] Eftekhar NS. Introduction. In: Eftekhar NS, editor. Principles of total hip arthroplasty. St. Louis (MO): CV Mosby; 1978. p. 1–7.

[5] Hoefle WD. A surgical procedure for prosthetic total hip replacement in the dog. J Am Anim Hosp Assoc 1974;10:269–76.

[6] Leighton RL. The Richard's II canine hip prosthesis. J Am Anim Hosp Assoc 1979;15:73–6.

[7] Lewis RG, Jones JP. A clinical study of canine total hip arthroplasty. Vet Surg 1980;9:20–3.

[8] Parker RB, Bloomberg MS, Bitetto W. Canine total hip arthroplasty: a clinical review of 20 cases. J Am Anim Hosp Assoc 1984;20:97–104.

[9] Olmstead M. The canine cemented modular total hip prosthesis. J Am Anim Hosp 1995;31:109–24.

[10] Olmstead M. Total hip replacement in the dog. Semin Vet Med Surg (Small Anim) 1987;2:131–40.

[11] Olmstead M, Hohn RB, Turner TM. A five year study of 221 total hip replacements in the dog. J Am Vet Med Assoc 1983;183:191–4.

[12] Montgomery RD, Milton JL, Pernell R, et al. Total hip arthroplasty for treatment of canine hip dysplasia. Vet Clin N Am 1992;22:703–19.

[13] Skurla CT, James SP. A comparison of canine and human UHMWPE acetabular component wear. Biomed Sci Instrum 2001;37:245–50.

[14] Hielm-Bjorkman AK, Kuusela E, Liman A, et al. Evaluation of methods for assessment of pain associated with chronic osteoarthritis in dogs. J Am Vet Med Assoc 2003;222(11):1552–8.

[15] Nelson JP, Glassburn AR Jr, Talbott RD, et al. The effect of previous surgery, operating room environment, and preventive antibiotics on postoperative infection following total hip arthroplasty. Clin Orthop Relat Res 1980;147:167–9.

[16] Gitelis S, Heligman D, Quill G, et al. The use of large allografts for tumor reconstruction and salvage of the failed total hip arthroplasty. Clin Orthop Relat Res 1988;231:62–70.

[17] Merritt K, Rodrigo JJ. Immune response to synthetic materials: sensitization of patients receiving orthopaedic implants. Clin Orthop Relat Res 1996;326:71–9.
[18] Milavec-Puretic V, Orlic D, Marusic A. Sensitivity to metals in 40 patients with failed hip endoprosthesis. Arch Orthop Trauma Surg 1998;117(6–7):383–6.
[19] Edwards MR, Egger EL, Schwarz PD. Aseptic loosening of the femoral implant after cemented total hip arthroplasty in dogs: 11 cases in 10 dogs (1991–1995). J Am Vet Med Assoc 1997;211(5):580–6.
[20] Schulz KS, Nielsen C, Stover SM, et al. Comparison of the fit and geometry of reconstruction of femoral components of four cemented canine total hip replacement implants. Am J Vet Res 2000;61(9):1113–21.
[21] Dearmin MG, Schulz KS. The effect of stem length on femoral component positioning in canine total hip arthroplasty. Vet Surg 2004;33(3):272–8.
[22] Fisher DA, Tsang AC, Paydar N, et al. Cement-mantle thickness affects cement strains in total hip replacement. J Biomech 1997;30(11–12):1173–7.
[23] Dassler CL, Schulz KS, Kass P, et al. The effects of femoral stem and neck length on cement strains in a canine total hip replacement model. Vet Surg 2003;32(1):37–45.
[24] Sangiorgio SN, Ebramzadeh E, Longjohn DB, et al. Effects of dorsal flanges on fixation of a cemented total hip replacement femoral stem. J Bone Joint Surg Am 2004;86A(4):813–20.
[25] Verdonschot N, Tanck E, Huiskes R. Effects of prosthesis surface roughness on the failure process of cemented hip implants after stem-cement debonding. J Biomed Mater Res 1998;42(4):554–9.
[26] Ebramzadeh E, Sangiorgio SN, Longjohn DB, et al. Initial stability of cemented femoral stems as a function of surface finish, collar, and stem size. J Bone Joint Surg Am 2004;86A(1):106–15.
[27] Orishimo KF, Claus AM, Sychterz CJ, et al. Relationship between polyethylene wear and osteolysis in hips with a second-generation porous-coated cementless cup after seven years of follow-up. J Bone Joint Surg Am 2003;85A(6):1095–9.
[28] Puolakka TJ, Laine HJ, Moilanen TP, et al. Alarming wear of the first-generation polyethylene liner of the cementless porous-coated Biomet Universal cup: 107 hips followed for mean 6 years. Acta Orthop Scand 2001;72(1):1–7.
[29] Iesaka K, Jaffe WL, Kummer FJ. Effects of preheating of hip prostheses on the stem-cement interface. J Bone Joint Surg Am 2003;85A(3):421–7.
[30] Li C, Kotha S, Huang CH, et al. Finite element thermal analysis of bone cement for joint replacements. J Biomech Eng 2003;125(3):315–22.
[31] Wykman AG. Acetabular cement temperature in arthroplasty: effect of water cooling in 19 cases. Acta Orthop Scand 1992;63(5):543–4.
[32] Stone JJS, Rand JA, Chie EK, et al. Cement viscosity affects the bone-cement interface in total hip arthroplasty. J Orthop Res 1996;14(5):834–7.
[33] Heisel C, Norman T, Rupp R, et al. In vitro performance of intramedullary cement restrictors in total hip arthroplasty. J Biomech 2003;36(6):835–43.
[34] Bishop NE, Ferguson S, Tepic S. Porosity reduction in bone cement at the cement-stem interface. J Bone Joint Surg Br 1996;78(3):349–56.
[35] Orr JF, Dunne NJ, Quinn JC. Shrinkage stresses in bone cement. Biomaterials 2003;24(17):2933–40.
[36] Shields SL, Schulz KS, Hagan CE, et al. The effects of acetabular cup temperature and duration of cement pressurization on cement porosity in a canine total hip replacement model. Vet Surg 2002;31(2):167–73.
[37] Baleani M, Cristofolini L, Minari C, et al. Fatigue strength of PMMA bone cement mixed with gentamicin and barium sulphate vs. pure PMMA. Proc Inst Mech Eng [H] 2003;217(1):9–12.
[38] Ciapetti G, Granchi D, Stea S, et al. In vitro testing of ten bone cements after different time intervals from polymerization. J Biomater Sci Polym Ed 2000;11(5):481–93.
[39] He Y, Trotignon JP, Loty B, et al. Effect of antibiotics on the properties of poly(methyl-methacrylate)-based bone cement. J Biomed Mater Res 2002;63(6):800–6.

[40] Weisman DL, Olmstead ML, Kowalski JJ. In vitro evaluation of antibiotic elution from polymethylmethacrylate (PMMA) and mechanical assessment of antibiotic-PMMA composites. Vet Surg 2000;29(3):245–51.

[41] Schlegel U, Sturm M, Ewerbeck V, et al. Efficacy of vacuum bone cement mixing systems in reducing methylmethacrylate fume exposure. Acta Orthop Scand 2004;75(5):559–66.

[42] Lahav A, DiMaio FR. Evaluation of a new power-operated PMMA vacuum mixing and delivery system for cemented femoral stem insertion. Orthopedics 2004;27(1):57–8.

[43] Geiger MH, Keating EM, Ritter MA, et al. The clinical significance of vacuum mixing bone cement. Clin Orthop Relat Res 2001;(382):258–66.

[44] DeYoung DJ, DeYoung BA, Aberman HA, et al. Implantation of an uncemented total hip prosthesis: technique and initial results of 100 arthroplasties. Vet Surg 1992;21(3):168–77.

[45] DeYoung DJ, Schiller RA, DeYoung BA. Radiographic assessment of a canine uncemented porous-coated anatomic total hip prosthesis. Vet Surg 1993;22(6):473–81.

[46] Schiller TD, DeYoung DJ, Schiller RA, et al. Quantitative ingrowth analysis of a porous-coated acetabular component in a canine model. Vet Surg 1993;22(4):276–80.

[47] Marcellin-Little DJ, DeYoung BA, Doyens DH, et al. Canine uncemented porous-coated anatomic total hip arthroplasty: results of a long-term prospective evaluation of 50 consecutive cases. Vet Surg 1999;28(1):10–20.

[48] Rashmir-Raven AM, DeYoung DJ, Abrams CF Jr, et al. Subsidence of an uncemented canine femoral stem. Vet Surg 1992;21(5):327–31.

[49] Walter WL, Walter WK, O'Sullivan M. The pumping of fluid in cementless cups with holes. J Arthroplasty 2004;19(2):230–4.

[50] Manley MT, D'Antonio JA, Capello WN, et al. Osteolysis: a disease of access to fixation interfaces. Clin Orthop Relat Res 2002;(405):129–37.

[51] Davis N, Curry A, Gambhir AK, et al. Intraoperative bacterial contamination in operations for joint replacement. J Bone Joint Surg Br 1999;81(5):886–9.

[52] Mills SJ, Holland DJ, Hardy AE. Operative field contamination by the sweating surgeon. Aust N Z J Surg 2000;70(12):837–9.

[53] Tietjen R, Stinchfield FE, Michelsen CB. The significance of intracapsular cultures in total hip operations. Surg Gynecol Obstet 1977;144(5):699–702.

[54] Lee KC, Kapatkin AS. Positive intraoperative cultures and canine total hip replacement: risk factors, periprosthetic infection, and surgical success. J Am Anim Hosp Assoc 2002; 38:271–8.

[55] Massat BJ, Vasseur PB. Clinical and radiographic results of total hip arthroplasty in dogs: 96 cases (1986–1992). J Am Vet Med Assoc 1994;205:448–54.

[56] Paul HA, Bargar WL. A modified technique for canine total hip replacement. J Am Anim Hosp Assoc 1987;23:13–8.

[57] Konde LJ, Olmstead ML, Hohn RB. Radiographic evaluation of total hip replacement in the dog. Vet Radiol 1982;23:98–106.

[58] Buchholz HW, Elson RA, Engelbrecht E, et al. Management of deep infection of total hip replacement. J Bone Joint Surg Br 1981;63:342–53.

[59] Garvin KL, Hanssen AD. Infection after total hip arthroplasty: past, present, and future. J Bone Joint Surg Am 1995;77:1576–88.

[60] Dowd JE, Schwendeman LJ, Macaulay W, et al. Aseptic loosening in uncemented total hip arthroplasty in a canine model. Clin Orthop Relat Res 1995;319:106–21.

[61] El-Warrak AO, Olmstead ML, von Rechenberg B, et al. A review of aseptic loosening in total hip arthroplasty. Veterinary and Comparative Orthopaedics and Traumatology 2001; 14:115–24.

[62] Bergh MS, Muir P, Markel MD, et al. Femoral bone adaptation to unstable long-term cemented total hip arthroplasty in dogs. Vet Surg 2004;33:238–45.

[63] Edwards MR, Egger EL, Schwarz PD. Aseptic loosening of the femoral implant after cemented total hip arthroplasty in dogs: 11 cases in 10 dogs. J Am Vet Med Assoc 1997;211:580–6.

[64] Liska WD. Femur fractures associated with canine total hip replacement. Vet Surg 2004;33:164–72.

[65] Mallory TH, Kraus TJ, Vaughn BK. Intraoperative femoral fractures associated with cementless total hip arthroplasty. Orthopedics 1989;12:231–9.

[66] Garcia-Cimbrelo E, Munuera L, Gil-Garay E. Femoral shaft fractures after cemented total hip arthroplasty. Int Orthop 1992;16:97–100.

[67] Moroni A, Faldini C, Piras F, et al. Risk factors for intraoperative femoral fractures during total hip replacement. Ann Chir Gynaecol 2000;89:113–8.

[68] Wu CC, Au MK, Wu SS, et al. Risk factors of postoperative femoral fracture in cementless hip arthroplasty. J Formos Med Assoc 1999;98:190–4.

[69] Zuber K, Koch P, Lustenberger A, et al. Femoral fractures following total hip prosthesis. Unfallchirurg 1990;93:467–72.

[70] Duncan CP. The do's and don'ts of periprosthetic fractures. In: Proceedings of Current Concepts in Joint Replacement. Orlando, FL, February 2002. p. 123.

[71] Pernell RT, Gross RS, Milton JL, et al. Femoral strain distribution and subsidence after physiological loading of a cementless canine femoral prosthesis: the effects of implant orientation, canal fill, and implant fit. Vet Surg 1994;23:503–18.

[72] Engh CA, Glassman AH, Suthers KE. The case for porous coated hip implants: the femoral side. Clin Orthop Relat Res 1990;261:63–81.

[73] Kallos T, Enis JE, Gollan F, et al. Intramedullary pressure and pulmonary embolism of femoral medullary contents in dogs during insertion of bone cement and a prothesis. J Bone Joint Surg Am 1974;56:1363–7.

[74] Otto K, Matis U. Changes in cardiopulmonary variables and platelet count during anesthesia for total hip replacement in dogs. Vet Surg 1994;23:266–73.

[75] Terrell SP, Chandra A, Pablo L, et al. Fatal intraoperative pulmonary fat embolism during cemented total hip arthroplasty in a dog. J Am Anim Hosp Assoc 2004;40:345–8.

[76] Liska W, Poteet B. Pulmonary embolism associated with canine total hip replacement. Vet Surg 2003;32:178–86.

[77] Freeman CB, Adin CA, Lewis DD, et al. Intrapelvic granuloma formation six years after total hip arthroplasty in a dog. J Am Vet Med Assoc 2003;223:1446–9.

[78] Marcellin-Little DJ, DeYoung DJ, Thrall DE, et al. Osteosarcoma at the site of bone infarction associated with total hip arthroplasty in a dog. Vet Surg 1999;28:54–60.

[79] Murphy ST, Parker R, Woodard JC. Osteosarcoma following total hip arthroplasty in a dog. J Small Anim Pract 1997;38:263–7.

[80] Roe SC, DeYoung D, Weinstock D, et al. Osteosarcoma eight years after total hip arthroplasty. Vet Surg 1996;25:70–4.

[81] Ansari MM. Bone infarcts associated with malignant sarcomas. Compendium of Continuing Education for Practicing Veterinarians 1991;13:367–70.

[82] Dubelzig RR, Biery DN, Brodey RS. Bone sarcomas associated with multifocal medullary bone infarction in dogs. J Am Vet Med Assoc 1981;179:64–8.

[83] Stevenson S. Fracture-associated sarcoma. Vet Clin North Am 1991;21:859–72.

[84] Sebestyen P, Marcellin-Little DJ, DeYoung BA. Femoral medullary infarction secondary to canine total hip arthroplasty. Vet Surg 2000;29:227–36.

[85] Warnock JJ, Dyce J, Pooya H, et al. Retrospective analysis of canine miniature total hip prostheses. Vet Surg 2003;32(3):285–91.

[86] Pooya HA, Schulz KS, Wisner ER, et al. Short-term evaluation of dorsal acetabular augmentation in 10 canine total hip replacements. Vet Surg 2003;32(2):142–52.

[87] Conzemius MG, Aper RL, Hill CM. Evaluation of a canine total-elbow arthroplasty system: a preliminary study in normal dogs. Vet Surg 2001;30(1):11–20.

[88] Conzemius MG, Aper RL, Corti LB. Short-term outcome after total elbow arthroplasty in dogs with severe, naturally occurring osteoarthritis. Vet Surg 2003;32(6):545–52.

Vet Clin Small Anim 35 (2005) 1233–1239

VETERINARY CLINICS
SMALL ANIMAL PRACTICE

Emerging Causes of Canine Lameness

Mark C. Rochat, DVM, MS

Department of Veterinary Clinical Sciences, College of Veterinary Medicine,
Oklahoma State University, 01 Farm Road, Stillwater, OK 74078, USA

A review of the recent literature reveals that most orthopedic conditions affecting dogs and cats are relatively well-described entities. Much of the current literature focuses on investigating new methods of treating these conditions or addressing the nuances of diagnosis or treatment. Nevertheless, new conditions are reported on occasion and, with the advent of the World Wide Web, international journals, and the commonality of international meetings, widespread reporting of emerging conditions has become much simpler and more common. Some of these conditions appear as single case reports and are rarely reported again, whereas others become commonplace. Emergence of a new condition may be the result of refinements in diagnostic testing or of our improved understanding of previously "established" pathophysiologies. New conditions may also reflect the rise in popularity of a particular breed. This article attempts to assemble into a single reference an overview of a number of recently reported conditions in which lameness is the presenting sign.

INFRASPINATUS BURSAL OSSIFICATION

Previously, conditions of the infraspinatus muscle and tendon have been limited to contracture of the tendon. That condition is well described and produces a characteristic gait alteration. Recently, the presence of mineralization within the bursal sac of the infraspinatus tendon has been reported in Labrador Retrievers [1]. Orthopedic examination reveals forelimb lameness localized to the shoulder. Focal pain is often present when the tendon insertion is palpated. The findings of synovial fluid analysis and arthrograms are usually normal. Arthroscopic examination of the shoulder often reveals concurrent pathologic findings of other discrete shoulder structures, such as the medial glenohumeral ligament and biceps tendon. Radiographic examination of the shoulder reveals singular or multiple mineralizations within the infraspinatus bursa and sclerosis of the adjacent humeral head. The mineralized bursa is best observed in the craniocaudal view. The presence of infraspinatus bursal

E-mail address: rocket@okstate.edu

0195-5616/05/$ – see front matter
doi:10.1016/j.cvsm.2005.05.003

mineralizations without concomitant point tenderness over the tendon in some cases suggests that not all infraspinatus bursal mineralizations are problematic.

Intralesional injections of long-acting glucocorticoid (methylprednisolone, 60–90 mg) or surgical resection of the mineralized bodies seems to be the treatment of choice. Of four cases treated by steroid injection, two resolved and two improved. Treatment with nonsteroidal anti-inflammatory drugs (NSAIDs) and rest appears less likely to resolve the condition. Of four dogs treated with NSAIDs and rest, one resolved, one improved, and the remaining two were surgically treated. Surgical therapy involves exploration of the infraspinatus bursa and tendon by a craniolateral approach. The mineralization is attached to the bursa and may be adhered to the tendon. In the three dogs treated surgically (one primarily and two subsequent to NSAID therapy), all three improved but none resolved their lameness. At this time, it is unclear whether failure to respond to surgical therapy demonstrates that surgical therapy for this condition is inappropriate or if the continued lameness is a function of other joint pathologic conditions.

INCOMPLETE OSSIFICATION OF THE CAUDAL GLENOID

Incomplete ossification of the caudal aspect of the scapular glenoid (IOCG) has been previously reported as an incidental finding in medium- to large-breed dogs [2,3]. It has been termed an *accessory ossicle* and can occur bilaterally. Recently, IOCG has been reported as a cause of lameness in dogs. Affected breeds include Rottweilers, Labrador Retrievers, German Shepherd Dogs, Border Collies, Russian Terriers, Doberman Pinschers, and Bulldogs. The age of affected dogs ranges from 8 months to 10 years, and there is no apparent sex predilection. Minor trauma is rarely reported, and the duration of lameness can range from 1 week to 1 year. Other proposed causes for IOCG include abnormal growth and osteochondrosis.

Physical examination of affected dogs reveals mild to moderate shoulder pain, especially with flexion, and regional muscle atrophy. Radiographic examination of the shoulder demonstrates IOCG in all cases (Fig. 1). Other known causes of shoulder pain, including osteochondrosis dissecans (OCD), biceps tendon disease, and supraspinatus tendon disease, can also be present on survey radiographs or arthrograms. Synovial fluid characteristics are typical of varying degrees of inflammation. Increased uptake of radio nucleotide during the bone phase of bone scans can be observed, but no soft tissue phase changes are reported.

Arthroscopic examination of the joint typically reveals an osteochondral fragment separated from the caudal margin of the glenoid by a 1- to 2-mm gap. The gap is filled with strands of fibrous tissue. The fragment is mobile when manipulated. Fragments that are not mobile under manipulation should prompt a thorough search for other joint pathologic conditions that would explain the shoulder lameness. Variable degrees of villous synovial hyperplasia and synovial fluid turbidity are also reported. Other pathologic findings,

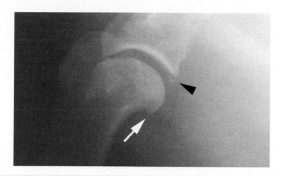

Fig. 1. Lateral radiographic view of a dog's shoulder. An incompletely ossified caudal glenoid (*arrowhead*) and secondary osteophytosis on the caudal humeral head (*arrow*) are present.

including the previously mentioned diseases and varying degrees of medial glenohumeral ligament injury, are also identified on occasion.

Histologic examination of caudal glenoid fragments reveals low-density cancellous bone bordered on three sides by fibrous tissue and on one side by normal hyaline cartilage (Fig. 2). The trabecular bone underlying the articular cartilage is poorly ossified or even cartilaginous, supporting the theory of an altered cartilage maturation process leading to incomplete ossification of the caudal aspect of the glenoid.

Arthroscopic removal of the osteochondral fragment and debridement of the adjacent edge of the glenoid result in resolution of lameness within 1 to 2 weeks

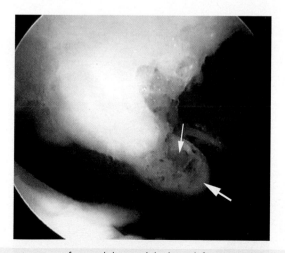

Fig. 2. Arthroscopic view of a mobile caudal glenoid fragment that has been partially debrided. The osteochondral nature of the fragment can be observed (cartilage surface, *large arrow*; subchondral bone, *small arrow*).

when IOCG is the only finding (Fig. 3). Lameness resolves in 2 to 4 weeks when IOCG is present in concert with OCD or when minor tears are observed in the medial glenohumeral ligament or biceps brachii tendon. When significant medial glenohumeral ligament injury is present, the extent of lameness usually improves but does not fully resolve.

ABDUCTOR POLLICIS LONGUS TENDOSYNOVITIS

The abductor pollicis longus (APL) muscle arises as a triangular muscle from the lateral radius, interosseous ligament, and ulna. Its tendon obliquely crosses over the tendon of the extensor carpi radialis and is enclosed in a synovial sheath. A small sesamoid bone is present in the tendon, where it crosses the medial aspect of the carpus. The tendon inserts medially at the base of the first metacarpal bone. The muscle serves as an abductor of the first digit, an adductor of the carpus, and a medial stabilizer of the carpus.

Straining of the tendon of the APL can lead to inflammation of the tendon and tendon sheath [4,5]. The resulting friction leads to secondary fibrosis and mineralization that impairs the gliding motion of the tendon and results in chronic lameness.

Dogs affected by APL tenosynovitis are usually large dogs of varying ages with no reported incidence of trauma to the affected limb. Chronic irritation of the synovial sheath, in some cases attributable to concurrent orthopedic disease in the contralateral limb, leads to inflammation and eventual stenosis of the tendon sheath. If the stenosis becomes severe enough, physical impingement of the tendon's gliding motion occurs in addition to the pain associated with more acute stages of the disease. A firm swelling along the craniomedial aspect of the carpal joint, varying degrees of loss of range of motion, and pain with passive

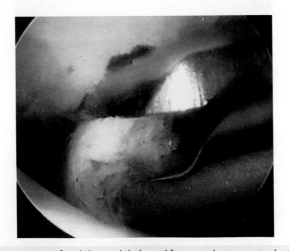

Fig. 3. Arthroscopic view of mobile caudal glenoid fragment being excised with arthroscopic rongeurs.

flexion of the carpus are present with this condition. Provocative testing (Finkelstein's test) used to diagnose a similar condition in human beings (de Quervain's tenosynovitis) does not seem to be of use in diagnosing APL tenosynovitis in dogs.

Radiographic changes include varying degrees of soft tissue proliferation, swelling, and bony proliferations along the tendon sheath. Radiographic changes do not seem to correlate closely with clinical signs. Synovial fluid characteristics are normal, and ultrasonographic examination of the region is reportedly of little value. Histologic examination of tissue excised from the synovial sheath demonstrates varying degrees of chondroid and osseous metaplasia and limited numbers of lymphocytes and plasma cells in the synovial lining.

In acute cases, injection of methylprednisolone into the tendon sheath is often successful. The distomedial radius and carpus should be clipped and aseptically prepared. A 24-gauge needle is directed proximally underneath the palpable tendon groove, methylprednisolone (20 mg) is injected, and the site is massaged. The joint should be immobilized for 3 weeks, and the treatment should be repeated if only partial improvement is observed. If the degree of lameness fails to improve significantly after one injection, the lameness continues after a second injection, or the condition is chronic, surgical debridement of the tendon sheath is recommended. After routine surgical preparation, a longitudinal incision is made over the distomedial aspect of the radial styloid process and fibrous and osseous tissue is resected from the thickened synovial tendon sheath until the tendon can freely move. A Robert Jones bandage (a bulky cotton bandage designed to compress the limb and reduce edema without creating vascular compromise) is applied for 5 days, and exercise is restricted for 3 weeks. Surgical intervention seems to be successful in most cases, but residual lameness can occur in some cases.

Loss of sensory capabilities, as a surgical complication, is common in human beings but does not seem to be a concern in dogs. Tenotomy of the APL is successful but may lead to medial carpal joint instability, especially of the intercarpal and carpometacarpal joints, and is not recommended.

DISPLACEMENT OF THE PROXIMAL LONG DIGITAL EXTENSOR TENDON

The long digital extensor (LDE) tendon originates from the extensor fossa on the craniolateral aspect of the lateral femoral condyle. The tendon courses distally through an extension of the synovial sheath in the muscular groove on the craniolateral aspect of the tibia. A thin fibrous band contains the LDE tendon in the extensor sulcus of the proximal tibia. The muscle of the LDE lies beneath the cranial tibial muscle. The distal tendon of the LDE passes under the proximal and distal extensor retinaculums around the hock. The distal tendon of the LDE divides into four separate rays that insert on the proximocranial aspect of the third phalanges of the second through fifth digits. The LDE is the primary extensor of the toes. Avulsion of the proximal LDE tendon has been reported as an atraumatic condition of young long-legged breeds, such as Great Danes and sighthounds, or in association with trauma [6]. Traumatic luxation of the LDE often occurs in conjunction with other injuries to specific structures around the stifle, including popliteal tendon rupture, lateral patellar luxation, and cranial cruciate ligament rupture. There are also reports of LDE tendon rupture secondary to abrasion by congenital lateral patellar luxation.

Displacement of the LDE tendon has been reported in conjunction with medial femoral malunion and stifle joint laxity [7]. Recently, a single case of bilateral displacement of the LDE tendon was reported. A 5-year-old Siberian Husky was presented for a bilateral pelvic limb lameness of 2 months' duration. No known trauma had occurred. The dog was being trained as a sled dog but could only perform short-distance training before becoming too lame to continue until being rested for 1 to 2 days.

Physical examination revealed bilateral pelvic limb muscle atrophy, no pain with manipulation of the stifle, and no stifle joint effusion. The range of motion in both stifles was normal, but flexion of the stifles with the limb loaded to simulate weight bearing resulted in an audible "snapping" sound that recurred when the stifle was extended. No drawer movement or evidence of collateral ligament instability could be demonstrated. Radiographs of the stifles were normal. Surgical exploration of the lateral stifle and proximal tibia revealed normal bony anatomy, but the tendon of the LDE could be easily displaced caudally from the muscular groove on the proximal tibia. Small holes were drilled through the cranial and caudal prominence associated with the groove, and braided polyester was passed through the holes and tied in a mattress pattern to simulate the normal fibrous band that traverses the sulcus and contains the proximal LDE tendon. The joint capsule, fascia, and skin were closed routinely. The limb was not externally immobilized. At the time of suture removal, the dog exhibited a normal gait but still had difficulty in rising. Joint range of motion was normal, and the previous snapping sound had resolved. Three months after surgery, the dog was sound and had returned to its original level of performance.

Although extension of the hock or excessive internal rotation of the tibia while the stifle is flexed may increase the tension on the LDE tendon and predispose it to luxation, the true cause of LDE tendon displacement in dogs with otherwise normal pelvic limb anatomy is unknown. Nonsurgical management of this condition may be successful in acute cases; however, generally, surgical creation of a prosthetic ligament to contain the LDE tendon in the muscular sulcus is successful and is considered the treatment of choice.

LATERAL FABELLA FRACTURE

Spontaneous fracture of the lateral fabella has been reported in Labrador Retrievers, Golden Retrievers, and Border Collies [8]. Most dogs are skeletally mature at the time of injury. The pathogenesis of this fracture is unknown, but it is speculated to occur because of imbalances between the cranial and caudal soft tissues that stabilize the stifle during range of motion. Specifically, imbalance between the gastrocnemius and quadriceps muscles may result in excessive or abnormal rotational forces around the stifle during range of motion.

The injury occurs during activity, but no specific traumatic event has been recorded. Dogs continue to use the limb, but stifle range of motion is restricted. These dogs are noticeably lame during activity, and the lameness worsens with activity and is exacerbated by rest. The injury usually occurs unilaterally but has been reported to occur bilaterally. Physical examination of the limb reveals point tenderness over the lateral fabella but no loss of stifle range of motion or joint effusion. Conservative therapy leads to fibrous union of the fabella, and clinical signs typically resolve in 10 to 12 weeks. Surgical excision of the fabella results in lameness resolution in 6 weeks.

References

[1] McKee WM, May C, Macias C. Infraspinatus bursal ossification (IBO) in eight dogs. In: Vezzoni A, Houlton J, Schrammer M, et al, editors. Proceedings of the First World Orthopaedic Veterinary Congress. Abbiategrasso (MI): Press Point; 2002. p. 141.

[2] Olivieri M, Piras A, Vezzoni A, et al. Incomplete ossification of the caudal glenoid. In: Vezzoni A, Houlton J, Schrammer M, et al, editors. Proceedings of the First World Orthopaedic Veterinary Congress. Abbiategrasso (MI): Press Point; 2002. p. 158.

[3] Olivieri M, Piras A, Marcellin-Little DJ, et al. Accessory caudal glenoid ossification centre as a possible cause of lameness in nine dogs. Vet Comp Orthop Traumatol 2004;17:131–5.

[4] Grundmann S, Montavon PM. Stenosing tenosynovitis of the abductor pollicis longus muscle. In: Vezzoni A, Houlton J, Schrammer M, et al, editors. Proceedings of the First World Orthopaedic Veterinary Congress. Abbiategrasso (MI): Press Point; 2002. p. 151.

[5] Grundmann S, Montavon PM. Stenosing tenosynovitis of the abductor pollicis longus muscle. Vet Comp Orthop Traumatol 2001;14:95–100.

[6] Piermattei DL, Flo GL. Luxation of the proximal tendon of the long digital extensor muscle. In: Piermattei DL, Flo GL, editors. Brinker, Piermattei, and Flo's handbook of small animal orthopedics and fracture repair. Philadelphia: WB Saunders; 1997. p. 574–5.

[7] deRooster H, Risselada M, van Bree H. Displacement of the proximal tendon of the long digital extensor muscle. Vet Comp Orthop Traumatol 2004;17:253–5.

[8] Houlton JEF. Fabellar fractures in the dog. In: Vezzoni A, Houlton J, Schrammer M, et al, editors. Proceedings of the First World Orthopaedic Veterinary Congress. Abbiategrasso (MI): Press Point; 2002. p. 110.

Vet Clin Small Anim 35 (2005) 1241–1245

ELSEVIER
SAUNDERS

VETERINARY CLINICS
SMALL ANIMAL PRACTICE

INDEX

Note: Page numbers of article titles are in **boldface** type.

0195-5616/05/$ – see front matter
doi:10.1016/S0195-5616(05)00102-6

Changing Your Address?

Make sure your subscription changes too! When you notify us of your new address, you can help make our job easier by including an exact copy of your Clinics label number with your old address (see illustration below.) This number identifies you to our computer system and will speed the processing of your address change. Please be sure this label number accompanies your old address and your corrected address—you can send an old Clinics label with your number on it or just copy it exactly and send it to the address listed below.

We appreciate your help in our attempt to give you continuous coverage. Thank you.

W. B. Saunders Company

SHIPPING AND RECEIVING DEPTS.

151 BENIGNO BLVD.

BELLMAWR, N.J. 08031

SECOND CLASS POSTAGE
PAID AT BELLMAWR, N.J.

This is your copy of the
CLINICS OF NORTH AMERICA

00503570 DOE—J32400   101   NH   8102

JOHN C DOE MD
324 SAMSON ST
BERLIN   NH   03570

XP-D11494

JAN ISSUE

Your Clinics Label Number
Copy it exactly or send your label along with your address to:
W.B. Saunders Company, Customer Service
Orlando, FL 32887-4800
Call Toll Free 1-800-654-2452

Please allow four to six weeks for delivery of new subscriptions and for processing address changes.